HowExpert Press

Pharm

101 Tips to Start, Grow, and Succeed as a Pharmacist From A to Z

HowExpert with Ann Klemz PharmD

For more tips related to this topic, visit HowExpert.com/pharmacist.

Recommended Resources

- HowExpert.com – Quick 'How To' Guides on All Topics by Everyday Experts.
- HowExpert.com/books – HowExpert Books
- HowExpert.com/products – HowExpert Products
- HowExpert.com/courses – HowExpert Courses
- HowExpert.com/clothing – HowExpert Clothing
- HowExpert.com/membership – Learn All Topics from A to Z by Real Experts.
- HowExpert.com/affiliates – HowExpert Affiliate Program
- HowExpert.com/jobs – HowExpert Jobs
- HowExpert.com/writers – Write About Your #1 Passion/Knowledge/Expertise.
- YouTube.com/HowExpert – Subscribe to HowExpert YouTube.
- Instagram.com/HowExpert – Follow HowExpert on Instagram.
- Facebook.com/HowExpert – Follow HowExpert on Facebook.

Table of Contents

Introduction

Congratulations! You've decided to become a pharmacist! Now what?

The answer depends on where you are in your journey. This book is designed to be all-inclusive for all steps on this adventure. Feel free to skip around depending on where YOU are.

There are a great many things commonly overlooked about this knowledgeable community of healthcare professionals. Did you know pharmacists are certified in all fifty states to give immunizations? They are the most easily accessible healthcare provider; over 90% of Americans live within five miles of a pharmacy. They are an underutilized, overlooked profession at times. After all, starting in 2005, *all* graduates from pharmacy school have a doctoral degree. Some schools initiated that curriculum change before then. Before that, pharmacists upon graduated had a Bachelor of Science in Pharmacy. Folks who have been practicing pharmacy since that time have more real-world experience than you can shake a stick at.

I have written this book through the lens of a middle-class white cis woman. I have written this for all audiences. I acknowledge my privilege here and now.

Overarching idea and message: all the things you didn't think about before making this decision.

None of this considers marriage, children, or life considerations of any sort.

Full disclaimer: I am also a self-help junkie.

Index of terms, alphabetically:

- AACP = American Association of Colleges of Pharmacy
- ACCP = American College of Clinical Pharmacy
- ACLS = advanced cardiac life support
- ACPE = Accreditation Council for Pharmacy Education
- ADME = absorption, distribution, metabolism, excretion/elimination
- APh = advanced practice pharmacist
- APhA = American Pharmacists Association
- ASHP = American Society of Hospital Pharmacists
- BCPS = board-certified pharmacotherapy specialist
- BLS = basic life support
- BOP = Board of Pharmacy
- BPS = board of pharmacy specialties
- CPA = collaborative practice agreement
- CV = curriculum vitae
- DEA = drug enforcement administration
- FDA = Food and Drug Administration
- HHS = health and human services
- HIPAA = health insurance portability and accountability
- HIV = human immunodeficiency virus
- HPSO = Healthcare Providers Service Organization
- ICU = intensive care unit
- ID = infectious disease
- IV = intravenous

- MPJE = multistate pharmacy jurisprudence exam
- MSL = medical science liaison
- MTM = medication therapy management
- MUE = medication use evaluation
- NABP = National Association of Boards of Pharmacy
- NAPLEX = North American Pharmacist Licensure Exam
- PALS = pediatric advanced life support
- PBM = pharmacy benefits manager
- PCAT = pharmacy college admission test
- PE = pulmonary embolism
- PGY-1 = post-graduate year one
- PGY-2 = post-graduate year two
- PharmCAS = Pharmacy college application service
- Pharm.D. = Doctor of Pharmacy
- Ph.D. = Doctor of Philosophy
- PMP = prescription (drug) monitoring program
- PSAP = Pharmacotherapy self-assessment program
- RCA = root cause analysis
- TPN = total parenteral nutrition
- USP797 = United States Pharmacopeial; Pharmaceutical compounding – sterile preparations
- USP800 = United States Pharmacopeial; Hazardous drugs – handling in healthcare settings

Lesson 1: Before Pharmacy School

Fit

Find the glass slipper

Tip 1 – Decide if the lifestyle suits you.

The first thing you'll need to do once you're considering pursuing pharmacy is to contemplate if the lifestyle is a good fit for you. Why do you want to pursue pharmacy? Think hard about this. What is at the root of your why? Having this notion rock-solid in your head will make the next eight years (and many beyond that) that much easier. Committing to a career in pharmacy will require a large investment mentally, emotionally, physically at times, and financially. The clearer you are on what you envision and where you want to make a difference, the more likely you are to succeed. That tenacity and grit will see you through the hardest challenges. Go in with your eyes wide open to everything happening in the field and your vision of the future.

1. Reflecting on your motivators will enable a properly informed decision. Pharmacy school and everything after will be a long hard slog without something pushing you through to the bitter end. Clarity and focus will prevent giving up. One useful tool is to ask yourself, 'why?' three times. Each time you ask yourself 'why?', it gets deeper into your motivators. Be honest with yourself.

a. Why do you want to practice pharmacy? Because you want to help people.

    i. Why do you want to help people? Because your grandma has diabetes, and you want people like her to understand their medications.

    ii. Why do you want to help people understand their medications? You want people like grandma to understand their medications safely.

        1. You are motivated to limit harm and maximize safety for patients.

    iii. Why do you want this pharmacy job in particular? You want money.

        1. Why do you want money? Because you want to travel more.

        2. Why do you want to travel more? You want to see the world.

            a. Global perspectives inspire you.

2. The market of pharmacy is a tough one right now. In the 1990s, there was a huge need for pharmacists. There were stories of pharmacists switching jobs left and right for the $10k sign-on bonus. People were starting to realize how knowledgeable pharmacists are and where they can contribute to the height of their degrees. The projected market in the '90s was for huge

pharmaceutical expansion in anticipation of Baby Boomers retiring. After those projections went public, schools realized how much money could they could bring in by offering pharmacy classes. After all, a lot of them already had medical and nursing programs. It's not that much of a stretch to add pharmacy. Once those programs started pumping out graduates, more schools opened, more pharmacists graduated, and the market oversaturated. The clinical roles of pharmacists have blossomed phenomenally, but the dispensing roles have imploded due to the unreasonable and often unsafe demands of large retail corporations.

3. I don't want to deter anyone away from the field that has my heart. My urge to reconsider is not a "you're not good enough to be in my field," thing. It comes from a place of "I've been in your shoes, and it is HARD but possible," thing.

4. Before you commit, evaluate the current trajectory of the pharmacy industry and decide where you fit in. With the cutback of pharmacists due to overabundance and the shortage of technicians due to lack of financial incentives, expect the two to meet in the middle. More places are utilizing tech-check-tech programs. Given advanced training, technicians can oversee each other more than ever, reducing the need for pharmacists. On the other hand, this frees pharmacists up to do more clinical, care-taking roles than in the past.

Tip 2 – Traits of successful pharmacists

Now, let's discuss successful pharmacists. Just as any path in life, there is no single way to be successful. Noting common traits is helpful. A good pharmacist can understand the minutiae of a single or combination of medicines in the context of a given patient. Balancing these two requires attention to detail as well as big-picture assessment skills. These pieces often fit together like a puzzle. Being able to see the forest through the trees is essential. Great pharmacists are strong academically, but also good with people. They need excellent written and verbal communication with nurses, doctors, and patients. I can't think of an avenue in life that does not call for strong communication skills. But when you're caring for the life of another human, this is an exquisite art.

1. A good pharmacist needs to be attentive, careful, focused, and detail-oriented. There is a big difference between 75mcg (micrograms) and 75mg (milligrams), but the visual difference (mcg vs. mg) is easy to miss. A patient could be 100x overdosed this way.

   a. The small picture details are not the only important thing, though. A strong pharmacist needs to keep in mind the bigger picture for all their patients. What are *THIS* patient's goals for their health? How can we help them achieve this? A 95-year old cancer patient may not hope to achieve 0/10 pain control. We can, however, help control their pain enough to see their granddaughter's wedding.

      i. Some patients have spiritual beliefs that may mean different care from what you think is best. Jehovah's Witnesses will not accept blood products such as transfusions and may be at higher bleed risks because that eliminates some of our treatment options. Muslim folk hold sacred the pig, which eliminates some porcine based medications from our treatment options. Treat the whole person.

   b. Assume the prescription you're working on is wrong. The minute you assume a prescription is correct, your guard will come down. This complacency will allow mistakes to slip through. Do not underestimate the possibility that it can and will happen to you.

2. Empathy and compassion.

   a. Empathy is an essential trait for any healthcare provider. There is a certain amount of empathy required to help a person in need. At the root of everything we do is a patient who is struggling. You do not know everything a person is wrestling internally. Patients may have financial challenges. They may not understand why people keep fussing over them. Caring for their health may not be a priority for them. You don't know the full lens through which a patient is looking.

3. Patience

   a. Have patience with your journey through school and after, patience with other teachers and healthcare providers, patience with patients, patience with the ever-changing landscape of the profession, good or bad, and patience with your own continued growth through this adventure of life.

4. Most good pharmacists are good at puzzles. Not jigsaw puzzles specifically, but seeing how seemingly unrelated things fit together. For example, it is common for patients to have delirium when they've been in the hospital for a long time. When a patient is delirious, it is necessary to address certain things that may seem irrelevant. With delirium, it is relevant to assess sleep cycles, daylight exposure, magnesium, new medications, discontinued medications for possible withdrawal-related symptoms, possible urinary tract and other infections, pain control, medical history (like dementia), and anticholinergic medication use. In their unique ways, all these things can contribute to delirium.

a. Anticholinergics are a category of medication that is known, especially in patients over 65 years old, to contribute to delirium. Their use, in general, is strongly advised against in this patient population for exactly this reason. The American Geriatrics Society maintains a list of medications called the Beers Criteria for potentially inappropriate medication use in older adults.

b. Keep an eye and an ear out for what is happening around you. Someone else's problem may be connected to the problem you're trying to solve. If not, it may become your problem shortly. If you are in a retail setting, keep that radar on when your technicians are at the window talking with patients. There will be keywords or phrases as well as, "they've been talking a long time," type of radar alarms you will develop if you're paying attention. Be aware when something is happening abnormally.

   c. Contrarywise, there *is* benefit to single-tasking as compared to multi-tasking. There is a sacred cone of silence that allows focus and careful concentration.

5. It is helpful to have a strong math and science foundation.

   a. For the most part, math is largely simple arithmetic, but doses must be accurate. Revisiting the example in number 1.a. again, 75mcg vs. 75mg. There is a factor of one hundred between the two numbers. You will need to know how to convert decimals. You will need to understand ratios and percentages. If there is 20g of fat in 100ml, how many grams of fat are in 250ml of lipid emulsion? Another way to ask the same question is: how many grams of fat are in 250ml of 20% lipids?

   b. The required science is complex. You will need a firm understanding of cellular biology, anatomy and physiology, and biochemistry. This scientific background is discussed at length ahead (number 5).

Vision

Tip 3 – Create a vision of your pharmacy school experience.

Spend time creating a vision of what kind of pharmacy *school* experience you want. Are you willing and able to move? Is a top school important to you? What, for you, is a deal-breaker? How do you feel about out-of-state tuition? Is there a specific path or experience you desperately desire along your course? How will your support network support you near or far? Would you do better with a large or small school experience?

1. Several different companies do studies to rank the colleges of pharmacy. They all review slightly different criteria. Look at the most current rankings and decide where these things factor into your decision making.

    a. US News[1]:

        i. The methodology of this company's ranking is based exclusively on surveys sent to deans, faculty, and administrators at each school. Their website indicates there was a forty percent response rate from the colleges surveyed.

        ii. The U.S. News results are the most reliable and most commonly cited. The pharmacy programs rely on these results to promote their programs as "top pharmacy programs."

        1. They have ranking guides for public health, healthcare management, PA, rehabilitation, veterinary, social work programs, and more.

b. Pharmacy Technician Guide[2]:

   i. The factors considered for this ranking include:

      1. 60% was based on NAPLEX pass rates for the previous four years
      2. 15% research activity
      3. 10% graduation rates
      4. 10% student-to-faculty ratio and faculty credentials
      5. 5% their discretion
      a. They acknowledge student rankings, extra-curricular activities, student organizations, and professional and personal growth opportunities to students.
      6. They indicate that the committee that devised this ranking did consider the results of the US News ranking discussed above.

c. College Affordability Guide[3]:

   i. There is a ranking of pharmacy schools that evaluates the cost to the students. They are specific (but not clear) on the criteria that their primary focus is affordability for average to lower-income students. They do not simply list all colleges in order of cost;

there are some excluded as they are considered outright "unaffordable."

    ii.   This ranking[4] evaluates for-profit vs. not-for-profit status, Pell Grant recipient rates, use of financial aid, ability to pay loans after graduation, etc.

    iii.   If cost is a big concern for you, it may be worth looking at their rankings. They are different from US News and Pharmacy Technician Guide rankings.

  d. QS Top Universities[5]:

    i.   QS analyzes worldwide comparison. If you are interested in training out of the country, this is a great perspective. However, a lot of the remainder of this book may be irrelevant. Transferring licensure to the United States from another country is not covered in this book.

    ii.   These rankings[6] are based on academic reputation, employer reputation, research citations per paper, and H-index (a way of measuring both the productivity and impact of the published work of a scientist or scholar).

2. Another important point to assess is where you feel you belong. I mean physical location and socially. Financial concerns need to be acknowledged but are not the only consideration. Embedded within the question of relocation is a sub-question about what type of social experience

is important to you. Who are you and who are the type of people with whom you want to be trained? If you have attended undergraduate school in your hometown, you will naturally feel more comfortable than if you had moved away. However, you identify racially, culturally, ethnically, or gender-wise, seek an environment where you feel welcomed for who you are. All college environments will be differing levels of diverse and inclusive. A lot of pharmacy schools will post the statistics of recent classes, in terms of grades, gender, undergraduate degree percentage, and diversity. You may get a better gauge of this during your interview. Please, whatever your cultural filter, take the time to make sure your school experience is a good fit for who you are and who you want to be.

Tip 4 – Create a vision of your pharmacist experience.

Spend time creating a vision of what kind of *pharmacist* experience you want. Do you know ahead of time that you have a specific interest within the field of pharmacy? Different schools excel in different educational experiences. If you have a specific vision, look for related keywords on their website. Ask questions about your specific interests at the interviews. Call or email and ask their faculty. If you don't have a post-graduation vision, skip ahead to chapter 4: Different Pharmacy Sites to Consider and then come back.

1. Are you perhaps interested in a dual degree? Some pharmacy schools offer dual degrees in many areas, but common ones include:

   a. MBA (Master of Business Administration)
   b. MPH (Master of Public Health)
   c. MHI (Master of Health Informatics)
   d. PA (Physician Assistant)
   e. Ph.D. (Doctor of Philosophy)
   f. Doctor of Jurisprudence (JD)

2. Do you know ahead of time you want to contribute to the fields of oncology, transplant, or emergency medicine? To cater to your experience during and possibly after school, look for schools with large academic hospitals attached. They'll be better suited to meet these training opportunities for you. Are you in love with rural, independent pharmacy? Outlying mushroom schools are more likely to have staff and educators with experience there.

   a. Mushroom (also known as a satellite) school: When a school's primary site wants to add students to their roster, they create off-site programs. They can connect with the primary site via online and through video. They rent room(s) at another school. These secondary sites are called 'mushroom schools.' For example, I graduated from the University of Minnesota program but attended the Duluth campus. Their motto is "one college, two campuses." Some classes, like labs, are taught separately. To avoid conflicting experiences, perceived preferences, or favoritism, classes taught on one campus are broadcasted to the other campus. Some are taught on the primary campus and some of the secondary campus but sent via interactive television to the other.

i.   Setting up education this way requires classroom availability at two different campuses and carefully coordinated schedules. It requires adequate technical support and equipment.

Research

Required classes

Tip 5 – Research your school(s)' exact pre-required classes.

There is a standard list of required pre-requisite classes for most programs. From school to school, there are some slight differences, but they are largely the same. Research your schools of interest and ensure you've met every requirement before spending time and money applying. A comprehensive description of many colleges is available on the PharmCAS[7] website, the centralized application service many colleges of pharmacy utilize. There is a school directory with information available about all available colleges of pharmacy, including a full list of pre-requisite classes. Please note, not ALL colleges use PharmCAS. This website lists website and contact information, class sizes, any satellite classes, which dual degree programs are available, if PCAT is required discussed at length in number 7), and what the deposit is once you are accepted.

1. The standard list will take at least two full-time years to complete. Minimum. These classes typically include:

   a. Biology 101
   b. Chemistry 101 and 102
   c. Organic Chemistry 1 and 2
   d. Physics
   e. Calculus
   f. Statistics
   g. Cellular biology
   h. Microbiology
   i. Anatomy and Physiology
   j. General sociology or psychology
   k. Economics
   l. +/- Biochemistry

2. Most colleges will require Chemistry 1 and 2 and Organic Chemistry 1 and 2. Biochemistry is, as you may notice based on the name, the glue that connects biology and chemistry. How does your heart continue beating and your muscles contracting? How does your heart know to rest between beats, and how do muscles know when to stop contracting? Electrolytes like potassium, calcium, and sodium drive all of these. Taking it one step further, how do medications affect all these goings-on inside the body? How can we manipulate the heart rate when a patient's heart is beating too fast? And how can we get muscles to relax when they can't stop contracting on their own?

   a. I'm going to take a moment here and give you the basic rundown to everything science. All the pieces and players need to be introduced one item at a time, but they all tie together. Are you ready to have your mind blown?

i. Chemistry one and two starts at the most basic level (chemically speaking) and introduces the tiniest components of human (and non-human) life. All living things are comprised of carbon, nitrogen, oxygen, hydrogen, and a few other atoms. Every atom has a positive, negative, or neutral charge. A difference of charges on one side of a barrier compared to another is called a gradient. *__These charges are critical for everything that comes after.__*

ii. Organic chemistry – the name implies the chemistry of life-forms. It explains how, when these molecules join up with different types of sequences and bond types, they make certain shapes. These shapes are determined by where the charges are within the molecule (edges vs. middle). The charges on everything cause them to interact with the environment around them continually. All these interactions are based on charges. Whichever molecule has the strongest charge gets the say in terms of shapes and interactions.

1. Our primary go-to example of this is water. Water is composed of two hydrogens and one oxygen. The hydrogens have positive charges, and the oxygen has a negative charge. The three particles come together forming

a V with the negative charge towards the bottom with an ombre effect; the charge is graded throughout the molecule. If there are two molecules of water, the two negative oxygens and the four positive hydrogens will not want to touch each other. Positive charges repel other positive charges, and negative charges repel other negative charges (some physics thrown in for good measure!). The oxygen of one water molecule will be attracted to the hydrogen of a second water molecule. They stack sort of like cups. This fluctuating charge attraction is how water cohesively sticks together and why drops blob upward instead of outward. Water *wants* to stay with other water because of the balanced attraction and repulsion of charges.

iii. Biology 101 introduces different pieces. It zooms out a few steps to show you how living creatures are made and their composition. Biology lays the groundwork of genetics and basic cell design. After all, everything living thing is comprised of cells.

iv. Cellular biology breaks down cell form and function. Cell bio describes the pieces within the cells, including:

1. Walls – how do cells keep certain things in and others out? Answer: proteins and charges. But the full understanding of these comes later

with biochemistry. The answer has to do with the difference of charges on one side of a cell wall to the other side. This difference is called a gradient.

2. Organelles – where is the energy of the cell made and stored? Answer: mitochondria with the aid of charges.

3. How do all these bits fit into the cell? Why are there so many bits? What is the function of each of the bits? Answer: too long to fit here, but you get the idea.

4. How do cells communicate with each other? If your leg is being chewed off by a bear, that is something your brain will want to know and devise a plan to escape. The message of the bear chewing your leg needs to get from your leg to your brain, and an escape route needs to be quickly and efficiently communicated back downward.

v. Biochemistry combines biology and chemistry you've learned, which you can gather from its name. At the molecular level, how are proteins shaped? Why do they behave the way they do? Proteins comprise a large portion of the body functions; proteins have a charge and continue to interact with their environment. Proteins and the charges of the molecules within them dictate the overall shape. There are a lot of proteins in cell walls. These interactions take us back again to cellular biology and how the cells keep things in and out. It impacts how energy is made, used, and stored in the body. This energy can be harnessed, too. Say, for voluntary muscle contractions.

vi. Anatomy and physiology class zooms out to explain what the body is doing with the cells and these charges. Anatomy is the study of where things are physically located in and on the body. Physiology tells us how body systems work in the body.

    1. Your heart continues to beat because of the gradients of potassium, calcium, and sodium. The cell walls maintain gradients and cumulative charges on one side of the wall or the other. The difference in charge on each side of the cell wall is the entire impetus of how the heart beats. These gradients are the impetus for how the heart knows to stop, rest, and recover between beats.

    2. Your voluntary skeletal muscles contract because of calcium gradients. But they need to be told when to start contracting and when to let go. These contractions and relaxations work entirely different than the heart, but both harness gradients for power.

vii.   Pathophysiology is the study of what things are not working properly when a person has this or that disease state. This class describes what is working wrong.

viii.   Medicinal chemistry, then, shows us how to take what we know about ALL these ideas together and how to enable the body to take corrective action. It stops the wrong things from continuing through the use of medicine. Pharmacy explains how we can manipulate the body to do something different.

3.   Not always required, but I *HIGHLY* recommend a medical terminology course sometime in your undergraduate coursework if you can. These courses are rote memorization. If you have this solid base before pharmacy school starts, it is one less struggle during that rigorous course load. Most pharmacy schools offer a [online] medical terminology course but taking it in undergrad will:

a.   Allow you to harness this understanding on day one of pharmacy school.

b.   Free up your pharmacy school electives for deeper and more interesting topics.

Pharmacy Schools

Tip 6 – Research your ideal school(s)

Research your pharmacy school options. Decide if you're willing and able to move for school. What are the pre-requisite classes specifically at each of your schools? Some no longer require the PCAT, but some still do. Research how many and which letters of recommendation each will require. There ended up being one school I wanted to apply to but didn't because they required one non-math, non-science teacher letter of recommendation, but the only one I'd taken in the past two years was Psychology 101 with 199 other students. Know if there will be problems like that before you start dedicating your time and financial resources to these applications.

1. Some pharmacy schools are full six-year programs. A six-year program means they don't require any pre-requisite classes; you go right into the pharmacy program, and all classes needed are part of the program. If they are a six-year program, you apply to the program before you do any classes. If your school(s) of choice are NOT six-year programs, you will need to apply to the program once you are far enough along in your undergraduate work.

2. There are benefits to completing a four-year degree before starting pharmacy school. A large percentage of students entering pharmacy programs have them simply because the number of prerequisite courses is high. This courseload is a comfortable load for four years. It's also a standard, accepted progression. Having a four-year degree increases your options and is a common milestone. Completing the full four-year undergraduate experience allows students to

mature mentally and emotionally. It allows for time to develop professionally.

PCAT

Tip 7 – PCAT

If a school you're applying to does require the PCAT, I highly recommend getting a study guide with some form of practice questions. Practice questions should typically focus on biology, chemistry, and mathematics.

1. PCAT[8] is the Pharmacy College Admissions Test. It's equivalent to the SAT or ACT exam during high school. Three companies come into play when discussing the PCAT.

   a. **AACP**: The test is issued and maintained by AACP, the American Association of Colleges of Pharmacy.

   b. **Kaplan[9]**: the leading test prep company. They do not sponsor the exam nor have affiliation with the exam itself. They are leaders in preparing students for this and many more standard exams.

   c. **Pearson**: the security company that hosts the test-taking sites, scores the exams, and is responsible for allegations of cheating.

2. PCAT process:

   a. Testing takes place at given sites on pre-determined Saturdays July through February. Registration is open April through the following January. The earlier you register, the more likely you are to get your preferred site(s) and date(s). If you register late, there may be extra fees. The dates and fee are all available on the PCAT website. Currently, registration for the PCAT is $210.

      i. During registration, you may opt to purchase practice writing and multiple-choice exams.

   b. Like the NAPLEX and MPJE [post-graduate, pharmacy board exams] process, first, you complete an application to sit for the exam. AACP will review your application and approve your application. Then Pearson will allow you to select your preferred site(s) and date(s).

   c. During registration, if your school(s) of choice are PharmCAS members, you can designate them to receive your scores electronically from AACP. Typically, this is the only method through which schools will accept PCAT transcripts.

      i. PharmCAS is discussed in-depth ahead. It is a centralized application website.

3. The PCAT measures basic scientific knowledge, math, verbal, reading comprehension, and writing skills; and overall critical thinking skills.

It is a computerized, 192 multiple choice questions and one writing topic exam divided into five sections. The five specific sections are biology, chemistry, reading, reasoning (math), and writing. Each section is scored independently and scaled into a 200-600 score. The writing portion is graded by two separate graders on a scale of 1-6 and then averaged. Then all five scores are calculated into an overall composite score between 200 and 600 using an average of the five sections. The 90th percentile is usually about 430.

4. Some schools may require a certain minimum score to be considered for admission. These minimum scores should be part of your research.

5. You may take the PCAT five times. If you feel you need to retake beyond that:

   a. You may need to provide documentation to AACP that supports your reasons for the retake.

   b. You may need to reconsider, at this point, if pharmacy is still a suitable path for you. These skills need to be solid. If you're struggling this hard this early, the rest of pharmacy school will be exceptionally difficult.

Planning

Letters of Recommendation

Tip 8 – Letters of recommendation

Decide who you want to write each of your letters of recommendation. Approach them PERSONALLY (if able) and ask them to write said letters. Diversify your letters as best you can; this shows the potential school how well-rounded you are. For example, a coworker, a teacher, and a mentor. There will likely be specific requirements, such as math/science, pharmacist, or non-math/non-science.

1. While deciding who to ask, consider how experienced people may be at writing influential letters. You want someone familiar with the process but someone who will have enough time to devote to giving a thoughtful letter. You want someone who knows you well enough to provide a meaningful letter.

2. There are lots of resources available online on how to write a great letter of recommendation if help is needed.

3.   For each person who will be writing you a letter, provide them with:

    a. Your ideas of your future practice (at least one area of pharmacy that inspires you).

    b. Your number 1 school choice.

c. The specific school for which you are asking a letter.

d. Let them know if there is something specific to discuss in the letter that would be helpful to you. For example, your grade in biology may not have been stellar, but you were there every day and showed up for help on the weekend, or they worked with you at Walgreen's for the last four years, or they have known you since you were three and you're reliable.

e. For letters of recommendation, the more information you can give the writer, the better. It shows the person writing the letter your passion, which in turn will show in the letter they write for you.

f. Realize that asking for this is not a sign of weakness. Almost everyone continuing school will need this type of letter. Flash forward 20 years into your career and envision how you'd feel if someone you've worked with for the last four years trusted you that much, they came to you at this critical, vulnerable time and asked YOU to write them a letter. Of course, you'd be happy to help them.

g. The more time you can give them to write the letter, the better.

h. Let them know the deadline. Perhaps tell people the deadline is one week sooner than it is. That way, you have extra wiggle time in case they procrastinate.

Personal Statement

Tip 9 – Personal statement

Use all your contemplation from numbers one through four to prepare this essay. Most pharmacy schools will have a certain number of characters or words for you to meet. Mine ended up being about a page and a quarter typed out. Note the length; there is a beauty to clearly and concisely stating your point. Your statement is the perfect opportunity to explain to your school(s) what you envision for your entire experience. It tells them why you want to be a pharmacist and why you want to attend their school. If you apply to more than one school, at *least* edit the bit about the school and why you want to attend this or that school. You need to unleash your passions and desires in this paper. Verbalizing things in this way will show pharmacy school(s) why it is important to you to pursue this. Putting your passions into words is an opportunity to highlight your communication skills, which are important in this field.

1. Have as many people review it as possible. It is a vulnerability to ask people to read how you've expressed your passions this way. Know that in the long run, you're doing yourself a favor. If there is a writing center on campus or you know an English major, have them edit it. Have one perspective from outside the medical community. Have another one from inside healthcare. Especially if you have access to someone who did or is attending the pharmacy school(s) you're hoping to

attend. This is an example of where the experience and connections come into play. Skipping ahead to the last two numbers of this lesson, you will find there further discussion on the benefits of working during this stage of your journey.

Application Process

Tip 10 – PharmCAS and applications

A lot of pharmacy schools use PharmCAS now, a centralized online application service. The idea is that students can upload all their necessaries like transcripts, personal statement(s), and letters of recommendation to one place and apply to multiple schools. It also provides a simpler process for colleges. Their website lists dates to be aware of, but it is up to you to ensure you meet all deadlines for any college to which you apply.

1. When you open your account on the website, you will need to fill out the information about the undergraduate college(s) you attended, and after that, transcripts can be collected. It is on you to initiate this collection.

    a. There are downloadable request forms for transcripts to print on their website. Print and complete the form and take it to your registrar's office on campus. If you are no longer located by campus, you may mail it in. They may require a fee but will mail the form with your transcript. Your PharmCAS account will indicate when it is received. Some [undergraduate] colleges may have the ability to send transcripts electronically.

b. If you still have pre-requisite classes to complete, you may still submit your application with an indication that your grades and transcripts will be added once available.

2. They will ask for your PCAT information (an admissions exam discussed at length in number 7). Whether you have already completed it or not doesn't matter. They can retroactively collect scores or collect them once you've taken the exam. If you have not yet taken it, when you do, you can indicate you'd like your scores to be sent to PharmCAS.

3. There is, of course, a fee for applying to colleges of pharmacy through PharmCAS. The fee varies according to the number of applications you'll be sending.

Interviews

Tip 11 – Dress professionally

Stating the obvious but DRESS PROFESSIONALLY. Being professionally dressed shows how serious you are. I recommend a full, professional suit for all genders. The more professional you appear to them, the more likely they are to see you as a serious candidate.

1. To boost the professionalism, bring copies of your application, letters of recommendation (that you have access to, some may be confidential, which is fine), resume, and personal statement.

Tip 12 – Come to interviews ready

When they offer you an interview, see if you can find out anything about the people who will be at your interview. It is always good to have questions; it shows your engagement. But if you ask questions that have easily accessible answers, it shows them you're not paying close enough attention or not trying hard. Look under the faculty pages and see if you can locate their area of interest or study. Which classes do they teach? Come up with a question about that area. Doing this may or may not work, but it is worth ten minutes of your time. If you can't, it provides a great conversation starter when you get there. The more questions you ask about them, the more flattered they are, and hopefully that will reflect in the ultimate admission decision.

1. If you can glean anything about who may be at your interview, look them up on the faculty pages. See what they research and teach. Would anything in YOUR experience relate to their interests and be something with which you can make a connection?

2. Even if you are unable to predict who will be there, ask them what classes they teach. Ask them what interests them about pharmacy and what they recommend for success in their class. Ask them if

there is anything in your application that concerns them or intrigues them. Ask them where they see the future of pharmacy and the future of this program.

3. Whether or not you can find information on the interviewer, come prepared to ask questions about the program, too. Look at the school website and bring a list of questions with you that are NOT covered on their website or promotional materials. It shows them you are engaged in what they are doing and genuinely interested in THIS school. Suggestions include:

   a. What are the leadership opportunities available to students?

   b. If you see this school offers a course/program that is unique, ask them WHY they think it is so important and how they provide their students with tools.

   c. How does the school help students succeed?

   d. What can they recommend to help your success?

Tip 13 – Be prepared for questions about you

Be ready for lots of questions about YOU. There are many resources available online, but common questions include:

1. What inspires you about pharmacy?

2. Why do you want to be a pharmacist?

3. Why do you want to attend THIS school?

4. Describe a situation you had when you disagreed with a coworker and how you handled it.

5. Pharmacy studies can be grueling. How are you prepared to handle this challenge?

6. Where do you see the field going in the future?

7. They may pose some moral or ethical dilemma and ask for your course of action. Such as selling over-the-counter needles without a history of diabetes.

8. How are you unique?

   a. Even middle-class white cis women can be unique. Are you the first person in your family to complete college? Are you the first in your family to advance to a professional degree? Are you from a lineage of pharmacists? Do you have a lot of pharmacy experience? Were you president of the pre-pharmacy club?

   b. YOU have something unique you are bringing with you. As Dr. Seuss has decreed, "today you are you, that is truer than true. There is no one alive who is you-er than you." Harness this.

Experience

Tip 14 – Get experience.

Get experience working in a pharmacy. Experience can make or break your decision. It gives you connections and folks to whom you can turn with questions. The easiest settings in which to get a job right off the bat is retail, hospital, or compounding pharmacies. Others like long-term care and home infusion are possible, too, but people don't typically think of those settings if they're not in the industry.

1. Complete disclosure: I'm one of those people who likes to know *EXACTLY* what I'm getting myself into before committing. I worked in a pharmacy for almost ten years before I started pharmacy school. I started at a retail pharmacy at age sixteen but wasn't sure I wanted to make a career out of it. After a while, someone reached out to me about needing technicians at a hospital pharmacy. I figured I'd give it a try. IT CHANGED MY MIND ABOUT EVERYTHING. The different settings and expectations were refreshing to me. I worked both for a while and then ultimately left retail to start college to pursue hospital pharmacy. I know many who have been successful in pharmacy school and after graduation, who did not have experience beforehand. It is possible. Knowing what you are in for, knowing the basic workflow and drug names, seeing how the pharmacists worked and talked, and seeing their biggest stressors changes your view. Experience is where the magic is.

2. Side note: When I applied to pharmacy school with ten years of experience, pharmacy school instantly knew I was serious. This amount of experience may or may not be possible for you, depending on your journey, and I understand that. But you'd be surprised how many people apply to pharmacy school, or any graduate work, with NO experience. In pharmacy school, having familiarity with the drug names and common dosage forms provides a huge advantage. For example, digoxin comes available as 0.125mcg and 0.25mcg doses only. On a multiple-choice exam, it can eliminate several options on a dosing question if one of them lists 75g.

   a. While some of my classmates were making and studying flashcards to the top 100 drugs to learn brand and generic names, I was able to focus elsewhere because of my experience.

3. If you don't have any experience working in a pharmacy and are unsure where to start, try a shadow experience first. If you are in high school or college, approach your advisor. In college, when you claim an intended major, you should be assigned an advisor that will be able to help steer you towards connections like these. If you are in the pre-pharmacy club, ask the advisor of that committee. If this isn't possible, call or physically go to a hospital or retail pharmacy and tell them you're a student considering pharmacy and you need a shadow experience. Pharmacists are approachable (but admittedly busy) and love to help pull you into their work. There may be disclosures or agreements that need to take place but, we LOVE welcoming new folks into our world!

a. Included in this topic is the notion of having a mentor. It is beneficial to you both to have a pharmacist you know and are comfortable enough to ask questions. A mentor is a role model to look to for advice and feedback. This dynamic can be spoken or unspoken. If you're too shy or self-conscious to ask, it's ok to observe from afar. The closer your relationship with the person, the better it will serve you in the long run.

Tip 15 – Working as a technician is different than working as a pharmacist

Realize that working as a technician is much different than working as a pharmacist. Watch the pharmacist. See how they spend their time. Notice what things on which the pharmacists are and are not focused. These should be hints to you. It is OK to ask them questions, too. People like to tell you what they know and where they're focused. They will likely be flattered that you're paying such close attention. Except for when it is CRAZY busy, I'm always happy to share my thought process with those who inquire. And I'm thrilled to act on these teachable moments as they present themselves.

1. One point I review time and time again with technicians and students [in a hospital setting] is our constant failure to SEND things in a time-efficient manner. Pharmacists verify dosing and appropriateness, technicians pull the medications, another pharmacist checks it for accuracy, technician delivers it. But in the end, if the nurse doesn't have it, the patient can't TAKE the

medication, and it doesn't matter how quickly we do all the other steps. I spend a lot of my day sending things and get frustrated when technicians and students don't pick up on this urgency.

2. Don't forget, knowing what you do NOT like in a work environment can prove just as valuable as knowing what you DO like.

Connections

Tip 16 – Start developing professional connections

Having connections inside the pharmacy field is critical. The pharmacy field used to be small. Now it's much larger, but it still involves a lot of "who you know." Much more than people realize.

1. Lay down foundations for professional relationships with pharmacists, technicians, and interns you meet along the way. You may or may not envision working at *THIS* pharmacy or even this type of practice after graduation. You never know who you may run into later when pursuing a new job. Or if your existing job hires a new manager. Or who could write you a fantastic letter of recommendation to pharmacy school or a job down the road. Six years after I graduated from pharmacy school, my department created a new clinical manager position. The person who got the position was a man with whom I had graduated from pharmacy school. I applied later at a long-term care pharmacy where the general manager was a student who did a rotation at my hospital. If

I ever went to the retail side, one of my co-graduates is a regional [pharmacy] manager for a large company. Having this metaphorical foot-in-the-door can be huge.

2. You don't know what projects may be coming down the pipeline for other facilities. Or sometimes, even your facility. The pharmacy managers and directors may play their cards close to their chest on certain projects until they're at a certain point. Knowing these projects is a big deal. You want people to reach a critical point in their project and realize they need YOUR help to make this vision a reality. For this to happen, you need connections.

Summary

Calendar of suggestions

Months before the first fall semester of pharmacy school	Action(s) needed		As early as possible
Minimum of 2 years	Ensure required classes taken/scheduled/planned		Start a personal statement
April (17 months before)	Start the PCAT process		Connections
April – October (17-11 months before)	Start the PharmCAS process		Research
July – September (14-12 months before)	Start letters of recommendation and transcripts (part of the application)		Experience/shadow
January (9 months before)	Deadlines for most applications		
September – February (12-9 months before)	Interviews		

Lesson 2: During Pharmacy School

Classes

Firm understanding of three particular classes, medication delivery, kinetics, and calculations, will set you apart. Rock-solid comprehension of this material, no matter which path you choose within the pharmacy field, will serve you well. These are described ahead in detail.

Tip 17 – Medication delivery class

1. Medication delivery class is important because no one else receives this training at the depth pharmacists do. Knowing how medications work molecularly and chemically is what sets us apart. Knowing how drugs are absorbed, dispersed throughout the body, metabolized, and eliminated from the body is our strength.

2. Included in this topic is the overarching concept of ADME. ADME refers to absorption, distribution, metabolism, and elimination/excretion. These four concepts are the cornerstone of pharmacy.

   a. **Absorption**. There are many, many dosage forms. There are tablets, capsules, granules, dissolvable tablets, buccal (cheek pocket), sublingual (under the tongue), solutions, suspensions, nasal, intravenous solutions, intramuscular solutions, subcutaneous (fat layer) injections, rectal and vaginal suppositories, patches, lollipops, creams, ointments, inhalers, nebulizers, ophthalmic (eye), otic (ear), and more. Depending on how a medication comes into a body, it is absorbed faster or slower, which means it can start working faster or slower. Other factors can influence how fast a drug works. Examples include if you've recently eaten, how fast your intestine pushes it through, altered anatomy, or something, (either food or another drug) that binds to the medication before it's been absorbed.

b. **Distribution**. After a drug makes its way into your bloodstream, it travels around the body. Depending on how charged (water) or uncharged (fat/oil) a molecule is impacts where in your body it will accumulate. Hydrophilicity and hydrophobicity impact how long a drug will be active in your body and areas of the body it will be able to access. For example, there is a protein barrier protecting the brain that can be difficult for medications to penetrate.

c. **Metabolism.** Normally, this happens in the liver. The body tries to make a molecule more polar (more charged) so that it can be trapped in the urine and eliminated through the kidney. Some drugs are active when they enter the body, and some are not. Additionally, metabolism can mean making a drug that is not yet active (pro-drug) into the active drug. Because metabolism commonly happens in the liver, any problems with a patient's liver can impact how quickly or slowly this happens.

Genetics can play a role in the speed of metabolism. Some drugs are not metabolized at all and eliminated.

    i.   The field of pharmacogenomics focuses on metabolism and is rapidly expanding. The medications currently utilizing pharmacogenomics is cancer therapies. Antidepressants and pain are the next most rapidly developing areas. Other fields are still under investigation and expanding.

   d. **Elimination**. Most drugs are removed from the body through two mechanisms, the kidney via urine or the GI tract via feces. Elimination is where some kinetics (next point) comes into play. Kinetics tracks these levels to optimize drug exposure but minimize patient harm.

3. Answers to these tricky questions and more are found in medication delivery class:

   a. Why is there no such thing as a caffeine patch?
   b. Why does acetaminophen have so many formulations?
   c. Why is it safe for a patient to be on oral and intravenous vancomycin at the same time?

Tip 18 – Kinetics class

1. Kinetics is crucial in neurology and infectious disease (ID), in both hospital and clinic settings. Antibiotics and most seizure medications have specific nuances that require fine-tuning dosages to ensure patients receive enough medication but

not too much. A lot of both types of medicine can have severe side effects when the levels are too high and are a huge disservice to patients when levels are too low. Some doctors, especially ID specialists and neurologists, do get training in kinetics, but this is where we can shine.

2. Some medications are dependent on specific body systems. For example, warfarin acts on and is metabolized in the liver. This medicine treats and prevents clots from forming for various reasons. If a patient has liver failure, their liver isn't working the same, and the dosing may need to be adjusted. Other medications, like meropenem, are eliminated through the kidney. As an antibiotic, if someone's kidneys are shutting down, the concentration of medication can get too high in their body. When meropenem is too high, it can induce seizures.

Tip 19 – Calculations class

1. Calculations. The math is typically basic but CRUCIAL. I cannot tell you the number of times I've been bogged down in minutiae but had to come back to basics. Math.

   a. Real-world example: The following image is a pediatric order I received at our hospital. All patient information has been de-identified for confidentiality purposes.

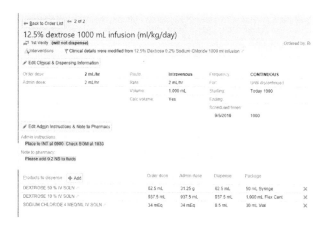

12.5% dextrose 1000 mL infusion (ml/kg/day)
⊡ 1st Verify (will not dispense)   Ordered by: B
⚠Interventions   ⚐ Clinical details were modified from 12.5% Dextrose 0.2% Sodium Chloride 1000 ml infusion ↗

✎ Edit Clinical & Dispensing Information

Order dose:	2 mL/hr	Route:	Intravenous	Frequency:	CONTINUOUS
Admin dose:	2 mL/hr	Rate:	2 mL/hr	For:	Until discontinued
		Volume:	1,000 mL	Starting:	Today 1000
		Calc volume:	Yes	Ending:	
				Scheduled times:	
				9/5/2019	1000

✎ Edit Admin Instructions & Note to Pharmacy

Admin instructions:
  Place to INT at 0900. Check BGM at 1030
Note to pharmacy:
  Please add 0.2 NS to fluids

Products to dispense ✛ Add	Order dose	Admin dose	Dispense	Package	
DEXTROSE 50 % IV SOLN ↗	62.5 mL	31.25 g	62.5 mL	50 mL Syringe	✕
DEXTROSE 10 % IV SOLN ↗	937.5 mL	937.5 mL	937.5 mL	1,000 mL Flex Cont	✕
SODIUM CHLORIDE 4 MEQ/ML IV SOLN ↗	34 mEq	34 mEq	8.5 mL	30 mL Vial	✕

Image 1: pediatric order for compounded IV solution

b. **Background**: When babies are new and early, their bodies can't control their blood sugar yet. When they are born REALLY early and small, they struggle to eat, too. Commonly they get their nutrition through an intravenous TPN, total parenteral nutrition. TPN goes directly into the bloodstream and provides protein, calories, sugar, and electrolytes until they can swallow breast milk or formula. Sometimes if they are medium early or small, they don't need all the things because they can drink SOME milk, or it will only be a day or two until they can. When that is the case, they get fluids such as the order above with more sugar than adults get. See on Image 1 how the ordering physician also asked the pharmacy to "add 0.2 NS to fluids"? This solution doesn't come premixed. We need to compound it. It is our job as pharmacists to calculate the amount of each ingredient to make this bag.

a. Reaching ahead to number 73, for pediatrics, always calculate twice and have another pharmacist check your work.

c. **Jargon**: in medical jargon, "NS" means "normal saline," which is 0.9% sodium chloride. 0.9% sodium chloride is 'normal' because it is roughly the same as what should be in a healthy body; it mimics the natural body environment. "Half NS" is half of that, or 0.45% sodium chloride. "One-quarter NS" is 0.2% sodium chloride and is what was ordered here.

d. **Calculating**: To solve this calculation, we need to know what 0.2% sodium chloride means. It means 0.2g of sodium chloride in each 100ml of solution. 12.5% dextrose means 12.5g of dextrose in 100ml of solution.
    i. We also need to know the ingredients we have to choose from to make the final product.

    ii. We carry 50% dextrose, 23.4% sodium chloride, and water.

e. **Sodium portion**: This type of math is called alligation. It is simple, but people don't trust how simple it truly is. Don't overthink it or make it more complicated. When subtracting, numbers do not go negative. Subtract the smaller number from the larger number.

% in products we have		% we want		Parts needed (subtract diagonally)	Number of milliliters
23.4				0.2-0 = 0.2	0.2 parts of 23.4%/23.4 total parts X 1000ml bag = 8.5 ml of 23.4%
	↘		↗		
		0.2%			
	↗		↘		
0 (water has 0% sodium)				23.4-0.2 = 23.2	23.2 parts of 0%/23.4 total parts X 1000ml bag = 990.5ml of 0% [water]
				0.2 + 23.2 = 23.4 total parts	

f. **Dextrose portion**: Repeat the same calculation with the same math.

% in products we have		% we want		Parts needed (subtract diagonally)	Number of milliliters
50				12.5-0 = 12.5	12.5 parts of 50%/50 total parts X 1000ml bag = 250 ml of 50%
		12.5%			
0 (water has 0% dextrose)				50-12.5 = 37.5	37.5 parts of 0%/50 total parts X 1000ml bag = 750ml of 0% [water]
				12.5 + 37.5 = 50 total parts	

g. **Total solution:** 8.5ml 23.4% Sodium Chloride + 250 ml 50% dextrose = 258.5ml additives

i. 1000ml total bag size – 258.5ml additives = 741.5ml water

h. To make this bag correctly, we added 8.5 ml 23.4% sodium chloride, 250ml 50% dextrose, and 741.5ml water. Boom.

Electives

Known path

Tip 20 – Elective choices

1. If you know exactly where you want to head after graduation, that makes selecting electives clear and simple. It should be obvious which electives will be most relevant. There may even be a suggested path or emphasis in place for you. For example, mental health, public health, or retail.

   a. I took a hospital elective that focused on the evidence-based practice of critical care (ICU) patients. We discussed several different facets of care like intubation, blood sugar management, addressing end-of-life transitions, anticoagulation recommendations, and post-stroke care. These areas all have in-depth studies and guidelines in place. We evaluated the history of the studies and why we care for patients in this setting the way we do.

b. A few of my retail cohorts took a dermatology elective. Dermatology is one area that patients may seek the recommendation of their (FREE) pharmacist before going into the doctor. They wanted to prepare for what they may encounter.

   i. Biggest take away: have the patient touch it. Do NOT touch it for the patient. If it blanches (turns white) when they touch it, start with hydrocortisone. If it doesn't, go to the doctor.

c. There are pediatrics electives available. As it turns out, this class focuses mainly on childhood diseases like sickle cell disease, childhood cancers, and taste of different antibiotics, and less on practical parenthood how-to's. If you have questions about what is or is not covered in an elective, you can typically reach out to the teacher/professor with questions or to see the last syllabus.

Unknown path

Tip 20 – If you're unsure of your path, diversify your electives

1. If you are unsure of what practice type you want to pursue after graduation, diversify your electives as much as possible. I took a diabetes elective, which was fantastic. I chose this because of the prevalence in society, and it still has a universal

applicability in pharmacy. Diabetes is a disease state that almost regardless of which practice site you pursue, you will almost certainly encounter. During this elective, we practiced what it was like to be 'diabetic' for a week. We checked our real blood sugar but then drew a fake number out of a bag, calculated how much insulin we would need based on our number and our meal, and injected ourselves (with saline; pretend insulin, not real insulin). We did this process four times daily for one week. It allows us fake experience but real-world-ish experience, allowing deeper compassion for future patients. It enables better understanding in the future while counseling or educating patients and to better answer their questions.

Both

Tip 22 – Electives with universal applicability

1. There are some electives/diseases that have universal applicability, like diabetes.

   a. As mentioned in number 20, some schools have emphases in place that can make elective selection simple. The University of Minnesota has a leadership emphasis. An emphasis like this is not exclusively for people seeking leadership positions down the road. There is a lot of personal and professional development course work in this emphasis as well universally applicable information such as conflict resolution, coaching others, and providing constructive feedback to others.

Tip 23 – Choose one elective because it's interesting

1. It is a good idea to add one elective that just plain interests you. For example, pharmacogenomics is largely delegated to oncology but is presently spreading into mental health. The sooner we can get to a treatment that works for *THIS* patient, the better we are serving them. More reasons to recommend an interesting elective:

   a. It may end up being more relevant than you anticipated.

   b. It may generate interesting conversations at interviews down the road.

   c. You may have a path in mind already set out, but life doesn't always take you exactly where you think it will.

   d. It is OK to enjoy your education. After a certain point, you may feel like you are doing what you are supposed to be doing, but it's OK to make your path into the professional world.

Curriculum Vitae

Tip 24 – Create and update your CV

1. Pharmacy is a field that doesn't use resumes for jobs; they use Curriculum Vitae. It's like a resume but much lengthier and more detailed. CV's should highlight your work and school experience. When deciding which to put first, use whichever makes you stronger. Include presentations you do during school, clubs and associations you join, the offices you hold, etc. Get yours started now. It's easier to start is now and keep adding to it, than waiting until the end and madly trying to remember all these things.

    a. Consider updating this after each semester. Frequent updates enables you to use it at a moment's notice for an internship or job opportunity.

    b. Be sure to include extracurriculars that are both pharmacy and not pharmacy related. Including the non-pharmacy ones will demonstrate your diversity. For example, if you volunteer at church or Habitat for Humanity.

    c. Extracurriculars helps to diversify your skill set, make stronger connections, and exposes you to more things.

Get Involved

Tip 25 – Get involved in groups

1. Join a group at school. Even if you choose not to pursue an office within that group down the road,

there are many benefits to this. It helps foster connections with staff and faculty of the college as well as your fellow students [including those above and behind you], it encourages your engagement with your school and the field, it bolsters your CV, and it broadens your mind. The exposure above and beyond the classroom is enlightening.

Experience

Tip 26 – Get real-world experience

1. If you don't have much real-world pharmacy experience yet, get some. It doesn't matter where or how much. Just get SOMETHING. It can be hard to work in addition to your course load. The money may not offset the MASSIVE student debt. The point is to get professional relationships started and familiarize yourself with drug names and basic processes. It will help you start putting pieces into context. Start figuring out what you do and do not like within the field. Start figuring out what you can and cannot tolerate in your long-term work experience.

    a. The easiest settings in which to get experience are a retail, hospital, or compounding pharmacy.

    b. If you do have a pharmacy job, bring what you are learning at school to work. Make one new brain connection each day in what you are learning at school and what you see at work.

       i.   Quiz yourself on mechanisms of action of the drugs you see.

      ii.   Quiz yourself on categories of the drugs you see.

    iii.   Quiz yourself on the side effects of drugs you see.

    iv.   What do you notice about patient interactions?

     v.   What did you learn, for example, in your cardiology section that you see being used in the real world?

c.   Tuition reimbursement may be available. Some companies will only provide tuition reimbursement if you commit to working at their company after graduation. A word of warning, though, the job offers you receive after graduation to meet this stipulation may not be what you expect. The company does not have to offer you something you WANT (location, number of hours, etc.); they simply must make you an offer to fulfill this requirement. If you choose not to accept their offer, you may have to repay the tuition money to the company.

d.   In the state of Minnesota, every intern hired has a precepting pharmacist. Someone they can go to with questions. I routinely emailed my preceptor throughout school, saying, "Hey, we talked about this thing at school, but I've never seen us do this. Do we do this?" Asking these questions provided a lot of interesting conversations.

i. I have several examples of questions I brought to my preceptor, but one example is when we talked about the prone positioning of patients that are intubated. Prone positioning means intubated patients spend some of their time lying on their fronts. Prone positioning puts pressure in different areas, opening up different places in the lungs. I saw this at a larger academic institution, but our hospital, it turns out, is too small for this treatment.

Setting up Rotations

Tip 27 – vary your site exposure

1. Vary your *site* exposure. Sign up for rotations at sites that are as varied as possible.

   a. Big urban hospitals, small independent pharmacies... my point here is to make sure your required sites are all different.

   b. Even if you know you want a specialty, there is still a benefit for a variety of exposure.

Tip 28 – Vary your experience exposure

1. Vary your *experience* exposure. For elective rotations, seek diversity. If you've worked at Walgreen's, don't select any Walgreen's rotations. Variety is important because there are SO many

different types of pharmacy. During these rotations is when you should try as many as different things as possible. Again, see chapter 4: Different Practice Sites to Consider if you're short of ideas.

a. By the time I was on rotations, I had already worked retail, hospital, IV compounding, and hospice. My elective rotations were industry (a pharmaceutical company's clinical trials division), MPHA (policymakers for pharmacists in our state), and a pediatric discharge counseling rotation. Do you know how difficult it is to explain the side effects of a medication to watch to the parent of a 5-year-old? How will a 5-year-old describe nausea or malaise to their parent to know it's the cause of a given medication? This experience was a huge eye-opener for me. This array of experiences allowed me to understand a broader scope of pharmacy.

Lesson 3: During Rotation Year

Curriculum Vitae

Tip 29 – Update your CV on rotations

1. While you are on rotations, continually update your CV. Take notes during your rotations on EXACTLY how you are spending your time. Document projects you work on, how many people and which types (technicians vs. pharmacists vs. nurses) come to your presentations, your presentation topics, what was your role at this practice site, who did you spend time with, etc. Add this info to your CV. Adjust your CV after each rotation, so it is fresh in your mind.

   a. Include on your CV future rotations; describe as "anticipated." This way, from December onward, when you start applying for residencies, jobs, fellowships, or post-graduate experiences, interviewers know what they can expect from you once you've completed all your rotations. Keep your CV at the ready for applications.

Setting up Post-Graduate Experience

Residency or fellowship

Tip 30 – The difference between fellowship and residency

1. The primary difference between residencies and fellowships is the context of practice. Residencies train pharmacists to provide care to hospitalized patients, clinic patients, and about being part of direct care teams. Fellowships train pharmacists to create new drugs and to be part of the manufacturing team. Residencies focus on clinical practice, like caring for patients who are in the ICU. Fellowships focus on training individuals to properly evaluate the design of and evaluate clinical trials to bring new drugs to the market. The context and monitoring you'll be doing, the things you're watching for, will be vastly different.

Tip 31 – Information about residencies

1. Residencies are available as PGY-1 and PGY-2 options. These two abbreviations stand for the post-graduate year one and post-graduate year two. These can either take place at the same facility or in different facilities. Some programs are applied to separately, and some are a combined two-year program. An administration program is commonly a two-year program from the outset. At the time of this authoring, residencies are not

required for pharmacists like they are for physicians.

a. The programs offered include inpatient hospital, MTM, and managed care.

b. The point of a residency is to give the resident three years of experience in a one-year time frame. It boosts your confidence. School provides the facts, and a residency provides context for using those facts.

c. Residencies run July 1st through June 30th of the following year, like medical residencies. The extra time allows new graduates time to focus on graduation and licensure. It builds in a little time for relocation if necessary. You may be able to catch a quick nap if you play your cards right.

d. Residency pay is roughly one-third to half of what a pharmacist makes. The benefit is the directed learning and added experiences to which you will be exposed. You will need to assess the cost vs. benefit for YOU to choose this path. There is a difference in pay between PGY-1 and PGY-2, but these numbers vary more based on-site and focus.

i. These experiences can include medication safety projects, MUE data (or medication use evaluation), management experiences, formulary considerations, and attending conferences.

ii. If the residency is ASHP accredited, there are specific criteria in place for experiences as well as feedback in each category. There will be ongoing project requirements and, typically, staffing requirements.

iii. Depending on your practice site after completion, some places provide loan forgiveness. There are restrictions, such as your new employer is a non-profit or rural practice site. Look into restrictions in your area before planning on this.

e. There are many rigorous and detailed requirements for residents and their experiences. Detailed, thorough guidance documents are present on their website for the most up-to-date information and requirements.

Tip 32 – This is the time to decide your post-graduate path

1. Decide if this will be your path. For most residencies and fellowships, the deadlines for applications are in December or January of your rotation year. Start laying that groundwork as soon as you know what you want to do.

a. Research local state and national meetings (ASHP) to learn about available residency programs. ASHP and others maintain thorough lists that are useful.

i. ASHP has a big meeting every December in the United States. This meeting is officially titled the ASHP midyear clinical meeting and exhibition. They are one of the leaders for residency advocates, particularly hospital-based. Their big meeting includes residencies and fellowship experiences.

1. If pursuing a fellowship, another fantastic resource is the IPHO (Industry Pharmacists Organization). Not all pharmaceutical companies attend ASHP midyear, so this organization will be more inclusive.

ii. Nationally speaking, a lot of residency directors and program representatives attend this conference to promote their programs. If you are considering a residency, even a local program, it is recommended to attend this conference during your fourth year. Some rotation sites even build in days off for interns to attend, knowing this is a big deal. This conference is a great way to talk with current residents for both networking purposes and to discuss real-world feedback on sites.

b. Submit appropriate paperwork on time. "Appropriate paperwork" includes transcripts, cover letter, CV, etc.

i. The cover letter is the post-graduate equivalent of your personal statement while applying to pharmacy school. Use that same passion and enthusiasm in your letter. Refer to personal connections if you've met the residency director or any pharmacists/technicians/residents/interns you know at the site. And as with any cover letter, highlight how they will benefit from having you there. Know what each site has to offer and what appeals to you most about it. Write about it in your cover letter and discuss it at your interviews. Be as specific as possible, so they can see you've researched *their* program. If you attended the ASHP midyear conference and especially if you talked with a program director, resident, or representative, discuss that in your cover letter.

ii. Your CV will probably be the same for each site if you are applying to more than one, but you should adjust your cover letter or letter of intent for each. As with your personal statement for pharmacy school, the purpose of this letter is to tell them why they are a good match for you AND why you are a good match for them. Focus on what you have to offer them that few others can.

iii. Don't cut and paste one cover letter to all your applications. If it has the wrong location name on it, it will not go well. Or if you go on about how excited you are for an opportunity that they don't offer. PLEASE double check and reread and triple check for accuracy.

c. There is a predetermined application process for residencies. ASHP has specific deadlines in place for applicants (early to mid-January). Once applications are finalized, sites can begin interviews. Once interviews are completed, sites enter their rankings for candidates, and candidates rank their choices for sites. All of these are then combined into what is called 'The Match,' whereby computer algorithms carefully assign based on these rankings.

2. Fellowships are typically applied to directly through the company.

3. Prepare for interviews mentally, emotionally, and financially.

4. If you are traveling for interviews, have the money saved away.

5. Most interviews will require a presentation of varying lengths. Decide your topic and begin creating it. These presentations are typically a case study encountered either while on rotations or intern experience.

6. If a site is out of the area for you, research interview dates, and where you can stay while you're in town.

7. At your interview, like pharmacy school interviews, ask lots of questions and be prepared for lots of questions about yourself.

8. Send follow-up emails to help them remember your interest in their program. Thank them for their time and consideration.

Connections

On rotations

Tip 33 – Collect references (people)

1. Collect business cards, LinkedIn connections, or whatever is hip these days while you are on rotations. Find some way to stay connected with pharmacists, technicians, and managers you meet. These people will be your most valuable asset at graduation. And in the future. Through your rotations, ask one or two people at each site if you may use them as a future reference. That way, when you decide which path to pursue, you have options.

Tip 34 – Always conduct yourself professionally

1. Always conduct yourself professionally. Yes, life does create obstacles, and preceptors realize you may be sick, get a flat tire, or have things come up. Be respectful in your interactions because every day is an interview during this phase. Be respectful in ALL your interactions; with technicians, nurses, doctors, patients, etc. You don't know how close they may be with your preceptor or what they will say when you are gone. You want them to miss you when you move on!

References

Tip 35 – Collect references (tools)

1. Here I mean tools and websites, not people. Take notes during your rotations on references you find as you go that are useful. Examples include dosing or dealing with specific challenges or disease states. After graduation, these references may be relevant again. Collect these references from everyone. Ask nurses which references they use for administration questions. Ask your preceptors, "what is one of the most valuable tools you refer to often?"

    a. For example, I have references for extravasation management, transitioning between anticoagulants, lactose-free drugs, gluten-free drugs, drug dialyzability, and others. I revisit these sites often enough that having a list is handy, but infrequently enough that I don't remember the websites directly.

    b. I keep mine in a physical book I keep at work. I have a page of notes entitled anticoagulation, a page for TPN's, a page called "where to find...", etc. Coworkers of mine ask to see my book on occasion, knowing I keep it handy.

Risks as a Student

Tip 36 – Double count all narcotics

1. Double count every narcotic that comes across your station. Even if someone else counted it already. Be sure that you are not at fault if something comes up short.

Tip 37 – Document exactly what you did

1. If you didn't document it, you didn't do it.

   a. Use every available technology for this — barcodes, notes, etc.

      i. Your school will have insurance to protect you against legal problems while on rotation. This coverage is limited. Be careful to what you expose yourself. While on rotation, most of what you do is directly overseen, so your exposure should be limited.

Lesson 4: Different Pharmacy Sites to Consider

Introduction:

There is more to this chapter than meets the eye. When a person unfamiliar with pharmacy thinks of a "pharmacist," they think of retail and possibly hospital pharmacists. There is much more out there than those two options. This chapter is an attempt to open your eyes to know all the wonderful places pharmacists can contribute to population health. There are pros and cons to every setting. When you are determining your path within pharmacy, be aware of all the pros, cons, and lifestyle requirements. For example, hospitals are open 24/7 and may require evening, holiday, and overnight staffing. Expect this to be part of the hospital package. Informatics, on the other hand, may require on-call time but most positions are salaried and therefore few holidays required.

As Elizabeth Gilbert so eloquently described in her book Big Magic[10], each place in pharmacy is a shit sandwich. Ok, she didn't say it quite like that. But that is how I read it. In context, what she was truly saying was in creative endeavors, each type of endeavor is its own flavor of shit sandwich. Being a writer versus painter versus underwater basket weaver will have different pros and cons associated with the lifestyle. It's easy to find the part you LOVE about each. It's the cons that can make or break your decision. And this is precisely why experience is critical before graduation. For creatives, you may have to hustle for clients or to

74

sell your work, but if you genuinely love the craft, you will make it happen. The same is true for every setting in pharmacy. And life in general. But that, friends, is a different book.

Hospital

Tip 38 – hospital practice typically requires a residency

1. Hospital is listed first because this is my practice type. I like *MY* hospital because it's big enough that we have pharmacists in many areas. It's also small enough that despite not completing a residency, I got hired on after I graduated pharmacy school and get to work decentralized areas anyway. Some hospitals do require a residency (especially large, academic hospitals), but mine did not. Full disclaimer: this is rare, and I had worked there for seven years before I graduated, including three before I got into pharmacy school. Hospital is a common option for those who decide retail is not their path. But it is not the only alternative.

Things to be aware of

Tip 39 – A day in the life of hospital pharmacy
1. What does my day look entail?

   a. Lots of consults from physicians who defer specifics to us on their behalf. These include but are not limited to kinetics, medication reconciliation, delirium consults, alcohol withdrawal protocols, anticoagulation dosing and education, PMP evaluations, and stroke review.

    i. With an acute awareness of the opioid crisis, states have banded together to communicate with each other. Currently, 42 states are exchanging data. The PMP[11] is "a tool to be used by prescribers and pharmacists to assist in managing their patient's care. It contains information provided by [state] licensed pharmacies and prescriber dispensers." It's a recording system for prescribers and dispensers (pharmacies) to see which prescriptions have been written and filled for controlled substances for a given patient. Patients who are 'seekers' may go to multiple doctors and multiple pharmacies to fill opioid or controlled medicines to an unsafe amount. This program is a method of working together nationwide to prevent this. We are sometimes asked by doctors in the hospital to evaluate a patient's history.

b. I spend a lot of time finding medication doses that have gone missing. It happens a lot. Like, a LOT.

c. Answering phone calls from nurses and doctors with questions about drugs, locating entries, the timing of medications, interactions, and much more.

d. Hospital pharmacy can be a shared work environment, depending on the size of a site. The amount of shared work vs. delegated work varies based on your level of training, but when I staff the central pharmacy, there are one or two other pharmacists. The work all comes from a pool that we're working on together. Sharing work this way can be good and bad.

Retail

Tip 40 – Patient contact

1. Patient contact. I hear time and time again how people are moved by the stories they hear and the patients they help. They develop lasting relationships with regular customers. Talking with patients allows pharmacists to check in with patients as to how their therapy is working for them and how their symptoms may be improving. Pharmacists can play a huge role in helping patients transition to their new setting with fewer interruptions in care.

   a. The importance of counseling cannot be overstated. Simple things like reiterating the route of administration for patients is easily overlooked by the non-medical trained folks of the world. I assure you, whatever you think people are not capable of, they will surprise you. Inhalers sprayed on the neck, reports of "chewy" tinfoil wrap on rectal suppositories, and "ineffective" birth control [oral] tablets placed into the vagina; the public will never fail to surprise you.

    i. What they teach in school is to explain things at a fifth-grade level. We can't assume that patients know words like or phrases like 'route of administration.' However, there is a fine line between full explanations and condescension. Don't patronize people; they don't want to be talked down to. It will invalidate your message and remove anything helpful you're trying to convey.

b. Connect with your patients, especially the regulars, on a first-name basis. Connecting with them this way enables a trusting relationship and fosters open discussion during counseling.

    i. Declining hours and extra demands of our profession are not the faults of the patient. The patient is the only reason we have jobs. As such, don't treat patients like they are a burden or an inconvenience. They will pick up on that, feel that, and it will immediately shut down any hope for open counseling or discussion.

    ii. Open, trusting conversation with regulars can lead to small things they can do to improve their health. When patients are collecting their insulin, ask them the last time they saw their ophthalmologist or podiatrist. Little things like this empower patients. They are told repeatedly by their doctors these appointments are important, but hearing it from their trusted, kind pharmacist can demonstrate that it IS truly important, and not just "one more" appointment.

c. Helping patients with copay cards, discount cards, manufacturer drug plans. It is important to note that "expensive" is relative. Every patient is in a different financial place in life, and we cannot assume what their [financial or other] priorities are. There are many websites available to guide these discussions. Many programs have [financial] restrictions in place, such as disqualification if they have Medicare as their insurer. One issue repeatedly encountered in our discharge setting is the cost of anticoagulants. We try to address these charges before the patient discharges, but we are not privy to every patient's full insurance information. Some insurance companies will give discounts for filling at a specific company's pharmacy, and we can't know all these nuances. Another factor is how long will this patient be on a given therapy. For example, there is a difference in taking medicine for atrial fibrillation (lifelong therapy) compared to a pulmonary embolus (PE; three months). Imagine a patient has a $200 per month copay for medicine they will take for three months vs. lifelong. The expectations of the patient and subsequent discussions change. Duration of therapy matters.

d. Courtesy and respect: If their prescription is delayed, always apologize. "I'm so sorry that took longer than anticipated, I wanted to make sure I wasn't giving you something that could hurt you," can go a long way to, again, foster a trusting relationship.

e. Trust your gut. Trusting your gut is a broad sentiment, and I mean this in several ways. If something seems off about a patient, ask them how they are feeling today. If something feels off about a prescription, call the physician. Again, we are the last step before *this* patient takes *this* medication, and we are the last step to ensure safety before it enters their body.

Challenges:

Tip 41 – Don't take it personal

1. Remember, if the patient at the window (or their loved one) has recently discharged from the hospital, they may be very angry, exhausted, or short with you. Know ahead of time that it's not about you. Waiting at the pharmacy, insurance frustrations, and fear for your or a loved one's health can make people cranky; they are not at their best when they see you. You are the only thing now standing between them and getting themselves or their loved one into bed at home for some peace and recovery. You cannot take these things personally.

Tip 42 – Metrics

1. Metrics. Metrics are a tough spot for retail. The current market shows little sign of improving. Big companies have rigorous expectations in place for numbers of prescriptions per day, the number of flu shots per day, and reports on patient medication compliance (based on how often they pick up a specific amount of medication). Companies have become exceptionally stingy on the number of technician hours, and pharmacists NEED these people to do their jobs well. They've buckled down hard on the number of hours of pharmacist overlap. If only one pharmacist is on staff, they're responsible for all the pharmacist-directed phone calls, patient questions, flu shots, and checking of medications. Also, some current law states that if the pharmacist leaves the pharmacy, the pharmacy must close. Bathroom breaks and food inhalation is difficult. Some retail pharmacies do close for lunch for this reason. When they do, I hear a lot of stories of pharmacists using this time to catch up, instead of caring for their bodies.

Tip 43 – Physical requirements of retail

1. Physical Requirements:

    a. Standing – lots and lots and lots of standing. Some pharmacists have indicated it's OK for them to use a stool, some companies may not allow it. When the pharmacy is busy and priorities are constantly shifting, it can be difficult to sit and continue performing.

b. Compression socks – highly recommended for long days of standing. Truly does make a difference. Additionally, comfortable shoes are your friend. Not only for retail but everywhere.

c. Lunch breaks are required by law but anecdotally few and far between. Many organizations and state legislatures are seeing this and trying to step in on behalf of safe working conditions. It is improving but has a long, long way to go.

d. Pumping:

a. Here and now is my only mention of parenthood in this book. Being a mother of three myself, I feel very strongly about this point. As difficult as it is to physically leave the pharmacy (discussed above), mom pharmacists who need to pump have expressed difficulty with this. If you work an 8, 10, or even 12-hour shift, one 20-minute pumping break is not enough to feed a baby or maintain mom's milk supply. Retail chains have gotten better about breaks, but this is exceptionally challenging and a sore subject among retail mothers. There are pumps now that allow discreet milk expression while working. Oxytocin, the hormone that causes milk release to begin expression, isn't produced at the same levels when you are working at the same time vs. staring dreamily into your baby's eyes.

e. Potty breaks – When you have to go, go. Easier said than done, yes, but this is your one and only body. Take care of it.

f. You are standing in front of a wall of windows. People can see you! Conduct yourself accordingly.

Clinic

Tip 44 – Clinic is slightly different from retail

1. This setting is like retail but located [physically] within a clinic building. Therefore, the pharmacist has access to hospital and doctor visit information. They can see the care team notes and see exactly what was discussed at the visit. Physical proximity makes accessing doctors for insurance changes or clarifying directions much easier. Because they can easily access the patient's information, they always have a full evaluation of allergies, accurate weight for weight-based medications, and kidney function for renally eliminated drugs. All of these advantages provide more accurate and safer patient care.

Clinical

Tip 45 – Clinical pharmacy is different from hospital and retail

1. Clinical and clinic pharmacists are, in fact, different; a *clinicAL* pharmacist means they have a specialty. There are SO many from which to

choose. Some specialties include infectious disease, HIV, oncology, TPN [total parenteral nutrition for patients who cannot eat], hospice, pain management, ICU, cardiovascular, psychiatric, surgical, orthopedics, eating disorders, transplant, emergency medicine, anticoagulation, neurology, and many more.

a. Pain management – this deserves a subcategory of its own. There are multiple ways of looking at pain management. Different kinds of pain need different treatments. There is surgical pain that we try to handle prophylactically, and there's palliative care, which is for more chronic or refractive pain. Palliative can overlap with hospice pain control but goals of care shift in this setting; our overall care is a little different. A separate discussion is that of addiction pain control. At the time of this writing, there is a lot of societal resources going towards combating the opioid crisis. Even though addiction and drug-seeking behavior are difficult to navigate, their pain still needs to be treated, and these patients still need to be treated with respect.

b. There are different paths to this job, just like every single life path is different.

Tip 46 – Fastest route to clinical is residency

1. The fastest route to becoming a clinical pharmacist is to pursue a residency after graduation. See the full discussion in Lesson 3: During Rotation Year

Tip 47 – Certifications beyond residencies

1. Certifications can be obtained to demonstrate proficiency or expertise in many specialty areas.

   a. BPS is the largest company but not the only sort of certification obtainable.

      i. The idea and benefit behind this certification are tying together a full knowledge base in patient-centered care. The initial certification represents minimum standards. Recertification (required every seven years) represents a pharmacist's commitment to ongoing professional growth. The BPS exams are designed to be rigorous, high-stakes exams.

      ii. Taking and maintain this certification is expensive. By design, the BPS only wants serious candidates. Some employers may aid in covering expenses for the exam itself or study materials. Some may or may not cover ongoing costs of maintaining the certification. Discuss this with your boss before you begin the journey.

      iii. They presently offer certifications in pharmacotherapy, oncology, MTM, ambulatory care, cardiology, compounded sterile preparations, critical care, geriatric care, infectious disease, nuclear pharmacy, nutrition support, pediatrics, psychiatric care, and solid organ transplant.

1. Pharmacotherapy, to make it equivalent to medical degrees, means you're specializing as a generalist.

2. Note this is not all-encompassing [yet]. Especially if you want to pursue an option not listed here, like anticoagulation or dermatology, you will need to find a different option. Other certifications and specialties exist, but due to space limitations, I cannot list them all here.

iv. National Commission for Certifying Agencies accredits BPS, which is a best practice arrangement. It is a voluntary submission that shows outside applicants they are serious, fair, and unbiased in their exams and certifications.

v. Because of this accreditation, they have no "teach to the exam" model. Their exams are all based on experience and application of taught material. To be clear, they do not TEACH the material; they presume you have already learned the material through pharmacy school and experience with or without a residency.

vi. For optimal fairness, each specialty has a specialty council comprised of nine pharmacists. Seven of whom have said BPS certification and two who have other or no BPS certifications. Each specialty council creates its eligibility criteria based on that patient population's experiential expectations. They are all slightly different like every patient and experience is expected to be.

vii. Several pharmacy companies offer preparatory courses for this exam. BPS certified pharmacists and other subject matter experts teach courses through APhA, ASHP, and ACCP.

    1. While some preparatory courses are online or in-person, the bulk of your studying is self-directed. BPS does not provide classes or materials to aid in the study.

    2. Most one- and two-year residencies expect their graduates will take the BPS exam after completion and will aid in study.

viii. There are two specific requirements for sitting for the exam. Requirements include a certain number of hours as a pharmacist (unless you've done a residency; this is exempt for residents). There is also a stipulation that direct patient care must make up a certain percentage of your time. As part of their accreditation through the National Commission for Certifying Agencies, they are required to disclose content outlines publicly. Each exam differs, but they have three to five domains, such as patient care, evidence-based practice, and population health. They are required to disclose the percentage each domain represents on the exam. BPS must disclose the weight of these domains. Spend your study time accordingly.

ix. Tips for studying for the BPS:

1. Look at the content outlines and plan your studying accordingly.

2. Having a study buddy helps tremendously.

3. This exam is presently offered twice a year. Where I live, it is in April and October. Evaluate the upcoming busy seasons of your life and plan accordingly.

4. Plan for the cost.

   a. If you fail, you may take it again. BPS will discount the cost if you take it again the next calendar year (2 cycles).

b. FASHP

i. FASHP = Fellow of the American Society of Hospital Pharmacists. According to their website[12], the purpose of this program is "to recognize excellence in pharmacy practice in acute and ambulatory care settings; and to grant recognition and to promote public awareness of pharmacists who have distinguished themselves within ASHP." Having this degree is an enormous honor in certain circles.

c. There are specific certifications one may obtain in other specific practices such as immunization certification and pharmacogenomics application.

Tip 48 – Clinical pharmacists can work in hospital or outpatient settings

1. These pharmacists can work in a hospital setting or a clinic setting. Some can do consulting work for pharmaceutical companies. We have in-house infectious disease pharmacists that look at de-escalation and serve as a reference for prescribers who are struggling to navigate allergies, culture results, and coverage (drug and bug combinations) while patients are hospitalized. Within our system, we have a separate clinic infectious disease pharmacist who focuses more on outpatient therapy. She spends time with infectious disease physicians performing follow-up, evaluations of adverse side effects, and following our HIV population.

   a. If interested in infectious disease, you may want to consider a PGY-2 specialty. It may also be relevant to consider a public health master's dual degree.

   b. One note to be aware of, our clinic infectious disease pharmacist spends a fair amount of her time working through cost and insurance barriers on behalf of patients. HIV meds can be considered specialty drugs and may not be covered easily. Some antibiotics, also, are exceptionally expensive.

Academia

Tip 49 – Academia

1. Pharmacists are needed to teach in pharmacy school, both in-person and online. Some, but not all, who teach pharmacy school classes are pharmacists. Having actual pharmacy experience brings a useful perspective to the class. It allows future pharmacists to gain insight from the things you have seen and learned. It allows teachers to bring perspective on what is relevant to the real world and what is not. Academia is an established career course with a lot of history. There is a large range of positions, especially in a specialized path like pharmacy. Some teachers are full-time, and some are not; some are tenured, and some are not. Of those that are not full-time, some continue practicing pharmacy.

   a. Depending on course load, additional responsibilities of professors may include:

      i. Research
         1. Research in academia can focus on the direct impact of medication use, abuse, and feedback from the actual public. Getting lay folks involved in pharmacy school classes is invaluable, both to the students and the public.
         2. There are many different research areas within pharmacy, too. Options include medicinal chemistry to SAPH, social and administrative pharmacy.

There is a huge range of areas for expansion within pharmacy.

ii. Precepting students on rotations

    3. Advising future generations of pharmacy students

iii. Proctoring exams

iv. Lots and lots of meetings

v. Admissions committees

vi. Updating lectures; this requires staying abreast of guideline updates.

vii. Office hours; answering questions for students directly

viii. Advising student groups. Depending on your experience and perspective, you can guide students seeking to follow a certain path into the pharmacy field.

b. Other things to consider if you choose to pursue academia:

i. Competition in this field can be tough. Ultimately competition between faculty can be damaging to the individual's work, the institution, and the field at large.

ii. Note if the institution you're looking at is unionized or not. Unionization alters the politics of the workplace.

iii. Get as many mentors as possible. Mentors are valuable everywhere, but especially here. The more perspectives you have, the broader and more applicable your work will be.

iv. Traditionally, academia is an exceptionally low turn-over career field. Know that the folks you're interviewing with that are already faculty will likely be your coworkers for a long time.

v. If you seek this path, graduate school [pharmacy school] will be the start of your career. Conduct yourself accordingly.

Industry

Background

The term 'Industry' refers to pharmaceutical manufacturing. It can mean both brand name drugs (new, first to market therapies) and generic drugs (drugs whose patents have expired, and multiple companies can sell them). There are separate companies for medical devices that require similar oversight by the FDA. Pharmacists are involved in several different capacities. This field requires a unique understanding of the law. There are many FDA regulations, application guidelines, and more. Pharmaceutical companies typically have legal departments that focus on meeting these regulations. This jargon includes GMP or good manufacturing practices; familiarize yourself. GMP is specific regulations promulgated by the US FDA. They dictate how and what is safe when creating medicine.

Different Options

Tip 50 – Industry will require fellowship

1. For this field, you will likely need to pursue a fellowship after graduation. Fellowships typically are two years. You complete both years at the same site or with the same company.

   a. You will need to be willing to relocate to where the fellowships and jobs are. Primarily east and west coast. There are fewer options available than residencies.

Tip 51 – Industry pharmacists can monitor trials

1. Pharmacists can help set up and monitor clinical trials.

   a. I did a rotation during my last year of pharmacy school in this type of setting. The company had a two-year program with one clinical scientist in each year of the program. They were studying anti-epileptics at the time. These medications require tapering *up* to start therapy and tapering *down* when stopping therapy. In certain clinical trial settings, you don't want patients to know if they are in the "treatment" arm or the "placebo" arm. This way, their answers will be more honest about side effects, effectiveness, etc. Creating taper schedules to disguise both real and placebo medications proved to be tedious and difficult! Crazy things like this are fascinating aspects of the field not often considered.

   b. Pharmacists (in this setting, also called Clinical Research Scientists) are also involved in making sure the study set up is correct and prompt. They regularly communicate with study sites to make sure all needed information is ready. They are the go persons to monitor study volunteer dosing. Being the go-to can include decisions on outlier volunteer approval and excluding or replacing volunteers as issues arise. Pharmacists monitor the overall study and documentation of every piece of the protocol as designed. The industry field is another area of pharmacy where if you didn't document, it didn't happen.

c. This setting relies on statistical analyses. Most companies will hire or consult actual stats experts, but the more you understand about your trial, the better.

Tip 52 – Pharmacists can answer calls from the public

1. Do you know that 1-800 number located on a drug's package insert to call when you have questions? They have pharmacists answering some of those calls. Common questions can include storage outside of the recommended temperature ranges, questions about side effects not reported, diluents for IV products, dosing outside of studied renal, hepatic, or weight-based recommendations, beyond-use dating, and more.

a. When we modify drugs in any way, we decrease their stability from the originally established expiration dating. Modifying the drugs and the subsequent change of stability is called their beyond-use dating. Modified can mean it has been repackaged (removed from the original container) or compounded in some way.

Tip 53 – Pharmacists can be MSLs

1. One more area within the pharmaceutical industry is MSL positions. MSL means medical science liaison. It's a person who has a therapeutic specialty (i.e., oncology or cardiology, etc.) and works for a pharmaceutical company providing education about specific medicines. They travel and educate physicians, other pharmacists, at conferences, and more. Historically companies didn't always provide education from trained healthcare professionals. Doctors and others became frustrated that these educations were coming from parrots, reciting what they'd +been taught and unable to engage in a meaningful discussion. Now, it's a great combination of clinical knowledge and industry that more and more companies are utilizing.

PBM (Pharmacy Benefits Manager)

Tip 54 – Pharmacists establish formularies

1. PBM means insurance companies. They hire pharmacists to establish formularies for the patients and companies they serve. Establishing formularies relies on folks who stay up to speed with new medications, existing options for specific

disease states, and current standard therapy guidelines. They also perform cost analyses and studies for their decision making. Another field jargon is 'place in therapy.' What else exists for that disease state? What do the medical guidelines currently recommend first, second, or third-line therapy to be? Where does THIS medicine line up with what already exists?

   a. Lots of places use formularies, not just insurance companies. A formulary is a list of medications insurance companies will cover or that hospitals will carry in stock, etc. It's impossible to carry or cover everything, so it must be defined.

   b. Breaking it down further, most insurance companies do not offer one single plan to its participants. There are typically multiple plans to choose from, and each covers things (medications, therapies, clinical specialties, etc.) slightly different. Individual plans decide what will or will not be covered.

   c. Examples of compelling indications can include cancer, pregnancy, and other options that were tried and didn't work.

Tip 55 – Pharmacists evaluate prior authorizations

1. Insurance companies have pharmacists review claims for patients that are NOT using the covered therapies. We call these prior authorization claims in the medical world. What it means is insurance companies decide (as described above) what will

and will not be covered. For example, you have a new PE [pulmonary embolism, aka blood clot in your lungs]. Your insurance company will cover warfarin and enoxaparin but will not cover rivaroxaban. In this setting, is there a reason it is better or safer for you to take rivaroxaban over warfarin and enoxaparin? Why do the doctors believe this is better or safer for you compared to the formulary medication? Reasoning in this way is called a compelling indication. Pharmacists review this information, the patient's case, the doctor's reasoning, and decide if they will or will not pay for this medication for this patient. These positions are becoming more remote-based [work-from-home] vs. office-based, which may be an influencing factor for some to pursue this line of work.

MTM (Medication Therapy Management)

Tip 56 – Pharmacists provide MTM

1. These pharmacists meet with patients and discuss their medications. They look at ALL the medications they are taking, including prescriptions, supplements, and over-the-counter medicines. They talk with these patients about how and when they take their medications (assessing compliance), discuss cost barriers, discuss problematic side effects or other barriers, and make recommendations to their physicians about therapy. Some have CPA's in place

(collaborative practice agreements) with physicians to go ahead and make changes on their behalf. Of course, all of this requires thorough documentation in the medical record. Because IF YOU DIDN'T DOCUMENT IT, YOU DIDN'T DO IT (number 37).

a. Some insurance companies are requiring MTM visits or give cost incentives for meeting certain parameters. Parameters such as a certain number of prescription medicines or have a certain number of diagnosed disease states. Studies have shown the overall cost savings in terms of medication use, side effects, hospitalizations, and general use of financial resources.

    i. This area can require cold calling patients to set up these appointments. Some may not realize it is a service covered by their insurance. It does involve a certain amount of salesmanship.

b. People who love the hands-on, patient interaction part of pharmacy can thrive in this setting.

c. One note to be aware of is that this requires a fair amount of documentation time. Again, if you didn't document it, you didn't do it. Have I repeated this enough yet? Documentation includes following up with patients and prescribers, billing for their time, and making notes of their recommendations.

Home Infusion

Tip 57 – Pharmacists work in home infusion

1. A fascinating and complex area of therapy where most lack familiarity. Home infusion is for patients who are sick enough they need intravenous infusions of varying flavors but are well enough that they don't have to remain hospitalized. Depending on how much someone can care for themselves (or their family can care for them), they may be able to do their infusions at home. Our home infusion department cares for patients on chemotherapy, TPN (total parenteral nutrition), antibiotics, hydration, and hospice related pain pumps. All of these require complex coordination with doctors, nurses, and patients.

    a. Fluorouracil is an essential ingredient to some chemotherapy regimens. This medication is infused [typically] over 46 hours, sometimes longer and occasionally shorter, but does not require ongoing hospitalization during infusion. Because patients will take this medication home while it continues to infuse, it falls under the purview of this department.

    b. Total parenteral nutrition can provide sustenance for people who, for various reasons, are unable to eat enough to keep their bodies nourished. Some are unable to eat at all. Trying to provide the right balance of calories, protein, sugar, and electrolytes can be exceptionally complicated but may vastly improve the quality of life for people who otherwise may fail to survive.

    i. Most patients on TPN are only on it while hospitalized and recovering from acute illness or surgery. Certain patients with chronic conditions need it long-term outside of a hospital stay.

c. The hydration patients we serve through our home infusion department typical*ly (but not exclusively) fall into two categories: hyperemesis gravidum and cancer. Hyperemesis gravidum is a condition of pregnancy where mama cannot stop vomiting. In a typical pregnancy, nausea recedes towards the beginning of the second trimester. Some women continue to struggle with nausea and vomiting throughout their pregnancy. Under circumstances of unrelenting vomiting, patients can become dehydrated, lose weight, and jeopardize their baby's health. Oncology patients suffer similarly. Due to their ongoing chemotherapy regimens, they have unrelenting nausea and vomiting, causing severe weight loss and dehydration.

d. There are various reasons and infection types that may require patients to be on long-term intravenous antibiotics. Osteomyelitis, an infection of the bone, is a common reason. Because this area of the body has little blood flow, it is difficult to direct antibiotics directly to it; therefore, the duration is typically 6-10 weeks. We've had multiple patients on amikacin, a different antibiotic used for tuberculosis and other lung infections. (Side note: this medication and several of the antibiotics we use require careful kinetics; see number 18). Typically, patients are on antibiotics for a much shorter duration than our TPN or chemo patients.

More!

Additional considerations

Tip 58 – Pharmacists work so many places

There are more subspecialties within pharmacy than I have time or capacity to describe. There are resources available online for a more in-depth conversation on these and many more. For demonstrative purposes, here are several more.

1. Compounding has become a specialty. Compounding can mean two different things, so clarification is important. There is sterile compounding, which means IV preparations going into a patient's bloodstream.

    a. Non-sterile: There are pharmacies dedicated solely to this process. Particularly hormone therapies.

    b. Sterile: an entire subcategory. As alluded to already, there are exceptionally rigorous requirements in place for places that provide sterile compounding. Many sites are undergoing costly construction because new guidelines are so rigorous. USP800 isn't exclusive to sterile compounding, but these changes severely impact sterile compounding procedures. The sterile compounding standard is USP797. If you're pursuing sterile compounding in any setting (a compounding pharmacy location, hospital, or home infusion, among others), familiarize yourself with these regulations.

    c. Legally, compounding can occur when a commercial product is not available. If an approved commercial product is available, pharmacies must select the commercial product to comply with FDA guidelines. Using commercial products over compounds is to prevent artificial cost inflation for patients and to protect patients' safety. Commercially available products are subject to harsh scrutiny during manufacturing. It is unjust to expose patients to additional risks unnecessarily.

2. Nuclear pharmacy

    a. Nuclear pharmacies and pharmacists dispense radioactive diagnostic drugs to hospitals and clinics. They take a radioactive compound (commonly technetium 99m or Tc-99m) and bind it with a drug to allow for administration. During administration, radiologists use special cameras to visualize where the radioactive medicine goes in the patient's body and how it moves around an organ. The purpose of these agents is to allow diagnosticians to visualize what is happening within a patient's body, usually a specific organ. For example, during a cardiac stress test, they will watch blood flow and perfusion to the myocardium to see if it is receiving adequate blood flow. The difference between this and, say, an X-ray is that this radioactivity demonstrates organ function as well as structure.

b. Nuclear pharmacists keep quite odd hours. Isotopes decay, which means the medicine will become less and less active over time. There is a finite timeline for preparation, delivery, and administration. Non-urgent doses are scheduled and administered during typical daylight, clinic-based hours. Based on these hours, doses will need preparation with minimal wasted time. Clinics usually open around 7 or 8 am. Timing requires overnight preparation. Hospitals with critical patients may require faster turn-around times with less notice.

c. Some pharmacy schools have electives in this field. This subspecialty does require special authorization or clearance with requirements for the number of hours with hands-on experience.

3. Investigational medicine

a. New drugs will always be needed. Society always moves forward. Additionally, we will always need to test new drugs. As discussed with industry, once new drugs are so far through the development process, we must evaluate safety and effectiveness in actual human beings. After limited clinical trials occur, these new medicines are given to select patients who are tracked and followed. As trials progress, we include more and more patients, which presents more and more diversity of responses. These trials include more and more patients, which allows researchers to see more and more interactions, side effects, and limitations of their drug. It is useful to have pharmacists tracking not only these things but also ensuring the patient is taking the drug as requested by the researchers. If the patient misses taking too many doses, their information becomes unreliable.

4. Informatics

   a. Internet connectivity continues to develop around the world. There is more demand for specialists able to link medical language with computer language. Both technicians and pharmacists are needed to create entries, link common languages, and ensure safe patient information storage. Translation worldwide requires a three-step process; translating one language (i.e., English, Chinese, etc.) into computer language and then computer language into a different language (i.e., French) to be understood worldwide. This field is expected to grow exponentially.

      i. Health systems have become more and more popular. Hospitals, clinics, and insurance companies all need to 'speak' to each other, use a common language, billing modalities, and security settings.

ii. Some colleges offer dual degree programs in informatics.

5. Research

   a. 'Research' can mean a billion different things.

      i. We will forever and always need new drugs for currently untreated or undertreated disease states. We, as a society, will always want better options.

      ii. There is a need for research on increasing compliance. Why are patients not always taking their medications as prescribed and how can we fix that? Do they lack the financial resources, understanding, prioritization, or something else? How can we empower them?

      iii. Ph.D. programs are for people who are interested in research as compared to PharmD programs. Having a PharmD will be useful. The curriculum for a Ph.D. is oriented differently compared to the PharmD curriculum. Curriculum and time frame depend on the Ph.D. program or educational goal.

6. Policymakers

   a. For our field to keep expanding, we need pioneers steering our trajectory at both state and federal levels. I'm making a generizationThis is a stereotype, but pharmacists enjoy putting their heads down and doing the thing. Whatever the thing is. We are not great advocates for ourselves. We need more unique thinkers to help us head in the right direction.

7. Management

    a. Pharmacies, like any other department, require managers. There are countless resources available for aspiring and current managers. There are two such books discussed in the additional reading section. Great managers give feedback and make their expectations clear. They praise in public but punish in private. They coach their employees instead of babysitting. Great managers can see and utilize the strengths of their employees for the benefit of that employee, as well as the department.

    b. One consideration for those pursuing management or director positions is the loss of clinical practice. Some pharmacists abhor this idea (for themselves), but good pharmacy managers must be clinically strong to make sound decisions for the department. The use or loss of clinical skills will depend on the role you will be taking. Know yourself and what you need for professional satisfaction.

Lesson 5: After Pharmacy School

NAPLEX and Law Exam

About the exams

Tip 59 – About the NAPLEX

1. First off, NAPLEX and law are two separate exams. Throughout your entire career, you MUST keep your initial state of licensure. You can reciprocate to some states without retaking the NAPLEX, but reciprocity is based on your original license. It must, therefore, never cease to exist. If you're looking at initially becoming licensed in multiple states, you indicate such on your application, and this indication is called a transfer. If you obtain, for example, three state licensures immediately at graduation, and later want to let one or two lapse, you may. You may select which one remains, but one of the three must always remain active.

   According to the National Association of Boards of Pharmacy (NABP)[13], "Each state board of pharmacy has a set of requirements that a pharmacist seeking licensure *transfer[1]** must meet before the board issues a license to practice pharmacy. Before applying for license *transfer[1]**, review the requirements for all states where you wish to *transfer[1]** your license. Some states

---

[1]*Emphasis mine.

require some combination of appearance before the board, a criminal background check, and a state transfer application. A few jurisdictions require a state law examination other than NABP's Multistate Pharmacy Jurisprudence Examination. Additionally, some states require that you pass the MPJE before submitting your licensure transfer application." It is your responsibility to know the requirements.

a. Note in the passage above the use of the word transfer. Highlighting the difference between 'transfer' and 'reciprocity' as follows:

   i. According to the Pharmacy Times in 2015[14], "When you originally take the NAPLEX, you have the opportunity to use the Score Transfer program to pursue a license in another state. Doing so allows you to become conveniently licensed in several states, each of which acts as your "original state." In other words, you can drop a state license at any time if you never want to practice there again. If you don't do Score Transfer and you want to obtain additional licensure, then you have to go through Reciprocity, which requires you to maintain your original state license throughout your career. For example, if you become licensed in Ohio, "score transferred" to North Carolina, and passed their MPJE, then you could drop your Ohio license at any time. With Reciprocity, you are stuck paying for your original Ohio license even if you know you will never move back to Ohio."

b. Reciprocity occurs after initial licensure. If you graduate from and begin your practice in Idaho and after three years decide to move to Missouri, you must maintain your Idaho licensure, renewing it as required by the Idaho board of pharmacy. You then take the Missouri MPJE but do not have to retake the NAPLEX to reciprocate your score.

Tip 60 – About the MPJE

1. The law exam is called the MPJE, or multistate pharmacy jurisprudence examination. This topic did not fall into my wheelhouse and was excruciating for me. Study, study, study. Lots of practice questions.

   a. The standard book for federal law is the purple Guide to Federal Pharmacy Law[15].

   b. Be sure you know what all needs to be in a Long-Term Care Facility emergency kit supply. This information and the next several bullet points are all laid out specifically in the Pharmacist's Manual[16], An Informational Outline of the Controlled Substances Act, available on the DEA website. Presently, there is an eighty-five-page PDF available freely on their website with clear terminology.

   c. Know what it means if a patient only wants to collect twenty of their forty-five oxycodone today. What happens to the remainder? Can they pick it up later? Does the remainder expire? Is the remainder forfeited? You need to know these answers.

d. Study the schedule classes of controlled substances. These titles refer to a specific jargon within the medical community. You need to know which medications fall into which categories. This information is laid out clearly on the DEA website.

   i. Schedule I means a given medication has little or no medicinal value and/or high abuse potential and is illegal.

   ii. Schedule II means a given medication does have medicinal value but has high abuse potential. These medications are legal but need careful use.

   iii. Schedule III[17] medications "have a potential for abuse less than substances in Schedules I or II and abuse may lead to moderate or low physical dependence or high psychological dependence."

   iv. Schedule IV medications have lower abuse potential than schedule III's.

   v. Schedule V is the lowest risk category and indicates medications that have maximum filling quantities. Worded differently, it means patients may not obtain more than a certain number of milligrams of certain medications at one fill.

    vi. There are specific record-keeping requirements for each category you need to be aware of, especially for Schedule II's.

Exam process

Tip 61 – Process for NAPLEX and MPJE

1. According to the NABP website, the board that oversees the exam questions and process, the application is a two-step process. First, you submit (to NABP) a non-refundable application fee. This fee is higher for certain states with additional eligibility requirements. Once you are approved to sit for the exam, you can purchase and schedule your exam.

    a. NABP = National Association of Board of Pharmacy. All the states have one joint program linking them for licensure and oversight. NABP tracks and documents continuing education (CE) credit for individual pharmacists.

    b. NAPLEX[18]:

        i. The NAPLEX is 250 questions. Two-thirds of which focus on "ensuring safe and effective pharmacotherapy and health outcomes," and the remaining one-third focuses on "safe and accurate preparation, compounding, dispensing, and administration of medications and provision of health care products."

ii. If you fail, you must wait forty-five days and pay the application fee again. There is a limit of five attempts to take the NAPLEX. If you do not pass during one of these five attempts, you are no longer eligible to become a licensed pharmacist. States may have mandates that with more than three failures, you will need to petition the state Board of Pharmacy to try again.

c. MPJE[19]:

i. The MPJE is 120 questions and is scored according to the following: 83% is pharmacy practice, 15% relates to licensure, registration, certification, and operational requirements, and 2% is general regulatory processes.

ii. If you fail, you must wait thirty days and pay the application fee again. There is the same maximum of five attempts before you are no longer eligible to become a licensed pharmacist. States may have mandates with more than three failures, you will need to petition the state Board of Pharmacy to try again.

Licensure

Tip 62 – Licensure is a separate application

1. This part seems tacked after graduation, but plan for it in the logistics of planning your post-graduation course. In addition to the two exam applications, you will separately need to apply to your state board of pharmacy to indicate your intentions of becoming a licensed pharmacist in their state. The licensure application gets lost in the shuffle of graduation but is an individual step that falls to you. Having attended a college accredited by ACPE (Accreditation Council for Pharmacy Education) is a requirement to becoming licensed. Assuming you have no hiccups before graduation, this does account for your "being of good moral character," a phrase embedded into the verbiage of many state boards of pharmacy. These two things, ACPE accreditation and "good moral character," are listed as requirements for successful licensure. The college will let the state board of pharmacy (BOP) know if there are problems that may inhibit your success as a pharmacist but still falls on your shoulders to physically apply for licensure.

Curriculum Vitae

Tip 63 – Continually update your CV

1. Keep this updated throughout your career. Every six months or so, update and reword your CV. You

may not mean to move jobs, but if something magical or inspiring happens to pop up, you will be ready.

    a. Add specific examples of what you've accomplished. Did you create new standard work? Did you pioneer a departmental book club?

Tip 64 – Services exist for CV revamp

1. If you need a serious revamp, there are several services out there that can review your CV with you. I've seen several pharmacist specific offerings on LinkedIn. Some will charge, and some will not. Some offer CV services only while others also offer coaching services if you're having trouble finding just the right job.

    a. CV services can be a non-traditional career path or simply a side job opportunity.

References

Tip 65 – Continue to collect references (people)

1. In this context, I am referring to people as references on your CV, not websites or tools. Collect references as you move throughout your career. I have asked people periodically if I can add them as a reference if/when I apply for a new job. I have about eight people currently who I keep as

references. On most job applications, you choose 3-5 of these people to list. If you know one of your references knows someone at the company you're applying to, use this to your advantage. If you're applying to an elite site and you have a pal who is a residency director or critical care specialist, that looks impressive.

Real-World Practice

Tip 66 – Respect HIPAA

1. Respect HIPAA. People get fired over this. Seriously.

   a. HIPAA is *WIDELY* discussed within the medical community but likely to be a lot of mumbo-jumbo to those outside of the community.

   b. HHS, the U.S. Department of Health and Human Services developed and continues to uphold this legislation.

      i. HIPAA's primary function[20] is to protect patient information. It allows patients access to information in their health records and to request corrections. It empowers them to know how their information will be used, to whom it will be disclosed, and why disclosure may be necessary. It limits the unnecessary release of information.

ii. It serves to keep violators accountable. *It is unlawful to disclose patient information without their permission.*

iii. For example, companies have fired employees due to leaking the names of hospitalized celebrities or famous athletes and their families.

iv. If you do not have a medical need to open a person's medical chart, electronic or traditional paper, you may not open it. That is made indisputably clear. As an employee, the action of logging into the computer system is us giving our consent to have our actions tracked. If I go into a patient's chart, the informatics team can see that and pull the record of my 'transaction.' Our computer system will create flags for informatics if I enter the profile of a neighbor or family member. They will be able to track my actions to determine if I had a medical need for this action. I have opened a chart of a person I know. Once I recognized the name of the person, I immediately closed their profile. I then asked a coworker to take care of their orders for me. Human resources did not approach me on this occasion, but if they had tracked my actions, they would have seen me open the profile, pause, and close it again. I didn't look at their medications, notes, or information.

Tip 67 – First orders verified is intimidating

1. I underestimated how intimidating it would be to verify the first few orders I verified on my license after graduation. That is one area that, unfortunately, we cannot get experience as students. Students can't be allowed to verify orders; there's too much liability. I didn't appreciate the gravity of accuracy until I clicked that "verify" button on *my* license.

Tip 68 – Handling chaos

1. Everyone has a different threshold for controlled chaos and uncontrolled chaos. Warning: upcoming equine reference. When things cross the threshold into uncontrolled chaos, and you start to panic, put your blinders back on and remember to focus on ONE THING AT A TIME. Horse owners use blinders for working horses or parade horses, so they don't see the horse next to them; instead, they focus solely on moving forward. There may be two calls on hold, three people in the drive-through, a nurse yelling at you, and four immunizations waiting. But you are only one person and can only SAFELY do what you can do. Our first and primary focus is to complete all tasks SAFELY. Be patient with yourself and don't quit.

Continuing Education (CE)

Tip 69 – Know your state's requirements for CE

1. Each state has numbers, specific requirements, and deadlines for continuing education. Know the dates and numbers for your state.

   a. For example, in Minnesota, the Board of Pharmacy (BOP) requires twenty hours of continuing education every two years. Our deadline is September 30th of even years. The BOP selects twenty percent of registered pharmacists to audit each cycle. From that point, you have sixty days to produce satisfactory documentation of all completed credits. If you are not audited, there is a simple affidavit and nothing more. Every state's procedure is different.

      i. Some states require a certain amount of law credits every cycle.

      ii. If you have a preceptor license, you may have specific CE requirements geared towards preceptor development.

      iii. If you obtain BPS certification, you can apply CE credit towards both, provided it is BPS approved CE. You will need to watch specific deadlines to ensure a given CE meets the timeline for both.

      iv. Initial certification and recertification in BLS, ACLS, and PALS all meet requirements for general continuing education.

   b. Don't wait until the night before to complete your CE (continuing education) or annual license renewal. You're adding unnecessary stress to your life. By cramming it all in for the sake of getting it done, you're not honoring the intention and spirit of usefulness for your patients.

Tip 70 – Resources for quality CE

1. Be OK with paying for quality CE. Don't get sucked into the garbage CE for the sake of getting it done. Obtain CE that will help you expand your practice, grow as a practitioner, and genuinely help you keep up to date on new medications, guidelines, and standard therapies. Do your patients and yourself the favor of high-quality continuing education. Some CE should cover topics that plain interest you, too.

   a. ACCP sells phenomenal continuing education, called PSAP (Pharmacotherapy self-assessment program). I have no financial affiliation to disclose, but theirs genuinely are much higher quality than the free stuff. I've done the free stuff, too. I have found, however, that if you are serious about professional development and personal growth, you will need to recognize this is one area in which what you pay for, you get.

      i. Your state branch of ASHP may provide lots of opportunities. The Minnesota branch is phenomenal. There are biannual meetings, endless online resources, and many events enabling networking and relevant topical discussions.

b. Our healthcare system subscribes to the Pharmacist's Letter and Prescriber's Letter. Because of our subscription, I get free CE from them, but I believe without it, there is a charge. Their education is less rigorous than ASHP but can keep providers up to date on guidelines and new recommendations.

c. Staying in touch with the alumni association where you went to pharmacy school can provide great opportunities, too. Many alumni associations host meetings with CE as a means of engaging students and graduated, practicing pharmacists. They may send invitations for meetings and presentations to alumni. It is valuable for the college to have alumni influencing the students as well as the students influencing the alumni. It enhances connections for both. It keeps alumni up to date on newer therapies and provides a real-world filter for students.

d. From time to time, go to conferences. Don't simply attend but engage in conferences. These opportunities have many benefits above and beyond the CE offered. They provide networking and connections and help you contribute meaningfully to the field. If you don't have the time or money to travel far, even attending state-based organizations is beneficial.

Tip 71 – Never stop learning

1. Never stop learning. Because you have graduated, the field does not stop moving. Everyone you meet can teach you something. By everyone, think patients, technicians, old and new pharmacists, interns, nurses, doctors, etc. By everyone, think EVERYONE. Don't be afraid to ask questions, too. It is OK to ask why someone is doing something. Be careful your questions don't come across patronizing. If you're genuinely trying to learn, typically, people are happy to explain how and why something is the way it is.

    a. Linked to number 72, next, have a list of people you can go to in different situations. People you meet in school, on rotation, or at your work. To whoever you are comfortable reaching.

Weaknesses

Tip 72 – Acknowledge your weaknesses

1. Acknowledge your weaknesses. If only to yourself.

    a. I know I'm weak on antibiotics. I know when I get these questions and orders that I need to double-check coverage, appropriateness, and dosing. I have a list of people at work that excel in this area, and I regularly curbside with them. I know, on the other hand, that people ask me questions about anticoagulation regarding timing, transitioning, and dosing when they struggle. We're all in this together. Help each other out. It's in the best interest of the patient that you are RIGHT, not that you knew the answer alone.

Tip 73 – Accept gray

1. There is gray in our black and white world. Physicians don't call us to ask questions about patients that are black and white. They know how to solve these problems. We are called and consulted when things are gray. Accept that.

   a. There is a fantastic book about this very idea by a phenomenal TEDx speaker and podcast host, Jonathan Fields, called *Uncertainty*[21]. If you need help accepting uncertainty in your life, try starting with this guy.

Connections

With Colleagues

Tip 74 – Build relationships with other departments

1. Build good relationships with other departments. Help and support them when you can. Consider this a future investment when you need their help for a project. You are not competing with others for your knowledge. Spread that shit everywhere. Helping colleagues helps you.

With Patients

Tip 75 – Treat patients with compassion and empathy

1. Treat patients the way you would want to be
    treated. Better yet, treat every patient the way you
    would want your grandma to be treated.
    Remember, you don't know everything about their
    history, their struggles, or what they have been
    through before they've made it to you.

    a. Compassion and Empathy are critical to
        patient care. See lengthy discussions in
        numbers 2.b. and 96. Pharmacists and
        healthcare professionals generally speaking
        seem to excel in this. That is, of course, a
        generality. But I think that's what draws us to
        the field of caring for others.

Mistakes

Prevention

Tip 76 – Preventing mistakes

1. An ounce of prevention is worth a pound of cure.
    Prevention can mean a lot of different things, but
    in this context, I'm referring to the
    answer/dose/problem to the question you are
    evaluating. When in doubt, look it up. When you're
    100% sure and it's a pediatric patient, look it up
    again. "Clarify before you verify!"

Tip 77 – It's OK to say "I don't know"

1. Don't be afraid to say, "I'm not sure but let me research that and get back to you." I used to believe a "good pharmacist" would know all the answers off the top of their heads. It turns out, you don't need to know all the answers, but you DO need to know how and where to find accurate answers quickly.

   a. That ongoing collection of references we discussed as students in number 35? Use that list for these types of questions.

Tip 78 – When in doubt, contact the prescriber

1. If you are unclear about the intentions of an order, contact the prescriber. Do not guess. They may give you a hard time (believe me, I've heard some horror stories here), but YOUR JOB IS TO ENSURE THE PATIENT'S SAFETY. That is our primary goal. If you are unclear about the intentions of a prescription, the patient may also be unclear. Maybe they know the answer. If an ER doctors write for eye drops for an injury or pink eye, sometimes, they don't include the duration. Ask the patient, "How long did the doctor tell you to keep using this medication?" If they don't know, make a clinical suggestion and document such. YOU are the only thing standing between this patient and safe vs. unsafe usage. Take this responsibility seriously. If you're struggling and can't come to a decision, remember:

   a. You must be able to sleep with your conscience.

b. If anything happens to this patient, you must defend your reasoning in a court of law. Did you do everything possible to make sense of this?

Tip 79 – Trust your gut

1. Never ignore your gut feeling. Not with orders, pharmacy in a broad sense, or life.

   a. Don't let anyone talk you out of a decision. If there are facts you missed the first time causing you to reconsider, that is OK. But your decision is based on experience and your gut. Trust that. If something feels wrong, investigate what is making you feel that way.

   b. Don't let patients bully you into something that causes you discomfort. If a patient doesn't like an answer (i.e., refusal to fill their narcotic early), it's because they know what they are asking isn't right. It helps to use the phrase, "it is illegal for me to..." Patients will typically back down when you subject the decision in question to legality.

      i. Do not jeopardize your license because a patient is mad you won't do 'X' for them.

      ii. Know and enforce with technicians what is pharmacy law and what is company policy. In other words, don't allow technicians to tell a patient something is the law when it's a policy and vice versa. Keeping this clear will prevent patients from using your words against you.

Handling Mistakes

Tip 80 – You will make mistakes; have support

1. You *WILL* make a mistake at some point. Have a strong network of support for when this happens. You are human, and I feel there is not enough discussion on these expectations in healthcare. I hope to change that.

   a. Related: don't judge others by the mistakes they've made. You don't know what they were going through. It could have been you.

   b. I'm going to share a story with you that makes me vulnerable. But I want to demonstrate my point and be my authentic self here.

   About a year after I graduated, I made a mistake that resulted in an RCA in our hospice pharmacy. RCA, or root cause analysis, is what our healthcare system uses to evaluate how and why mistakes happen. It is an in-depth investigation into the specific circumstances of an error and what can be done differently in the future to prevent something similar from happening again. In this story, I dispensed the wrong concentration of morphine solution. The patient was new to hospice and had been on morphine leading up to his hospice admission.

He was on morphine 10mg/5ml solution. The script written by the physician was for this strength. The error stemmed from the fact that our standard concentration for hospice patients is 100mg/5ml. The legal description of these two solutions is as written here. But there is a BIG difference. Remember that thing at the beginning where we said how successful pharmacists pay close attention to detail? I failed here.

My co-pharmacist and I both noted the nurse had requested 180 milliliters, and our standard bottle size is 30ml. Sending three bottles is a HUGE amount of drug. We both separately called the hospice nurse to verify they wanted 180ml, not realizing the other had called. *What we both failed to notice was the difference in concentration.* Our standard, when creating labels for hospice pain medications, is to list both numbers of milligrams and milliliters. Both these numbers were correct mathematically speaking.

i.   10mg= 5ml vs. 10mg = 0.1ml

Once it was delivered, the patient even called, and I spoke to him. He was confused about the difference between the volume he HAD been taking and what was on this label. I verified the number of milligrams and the number of milliliters but STILL DIDN'T SEE A DIFFERENT CONCENTRATION. I misunderstood his question about the number of milligrams compared to the number of milliliters.

I heard nothing more about this patient or this prescription until two weeks later. My supervisor asked if I remembered it and pointed out we dispensed the wrong thing. My heart sunk into my stomach, and my first question was, "was the patient harmed? Is he OK?" Yes, he was OK but hadn't taken any morphine because he was really worried about the difference from what he had in the past to what he got this time. He was smart enough to realize they didn't look the same. The patient trusted his gut.

However, his partner was admitted to the hospital because, as it turned out, she had been pillaging his stash, and she overdosed. She had a two- or three-day admission and was ultimately OK. But that in no way makes my error OK.

The RCA progressed. The RCA meeting itself involved a mediator, security, the next two supervisors above me from the pharmacy, the hospice nurse involved, the hospice physician involved, another hospice representative, and our two folks who specialize in mediating and resolving patient safety concerns. Everyone got a chance to explain what barriers prevented accuracy, and collectively, we brainstormed what, at each stage, what we can do differently next time. It was exceptionally stressful, but I quadruple-check all narcotics now. Additionally, our system added a step whereby we now barcode scan our narcotics. We had that in place already for non-narcotics but made it a priority to expedite a solution for narcotics as well.

Tip 81 – Acknowledge when you've made a mistake

1. When you do make a mistake, come clean as soon as you realize it. Acknowledge it to the nurse (if applicable), doctor, patient, and your boss. AND WITH YOURSELF. It may have happened as a matter of circumstances but acknowledge your shortcomings in the situation.

Challenges in Pharmacy

Tip 82 – Shortages are a challenge

1. Medicine shortages are a struggle for EVERY area of pharmacy and a complicated topic. There are several reasons this is happening.

    a. The FDA regulations in the United States is more rigorous than any other country. Given these steep standards, it can be difficult for drug manufacturers to meet the fluctuating demands of the market.

        i. Fluctuations occur for many reasons. Sometimes prescribing habits change. Perhaps new studies or guidelines are released that impact the use of one drug over others. If there is a shortage of one medication, all pharmacies across the globe may increase the demand for a different drug as a substitute. Then that company may have to increase production and run into another shortage problem.

ii. Raw materials shortages can be at fault. As the global climate changes, it becomes more and more difficult to meet the criteria for suitable goods.

iii. Rigorous FDA demands, combined with the expectations of patients globally, contribute, as well. See further discussion in the Industry section of Lesson 4.

Tip 83 – Cost is a challenge

1. The cost of medications to patients and pharmacies are a huge difficulty. Due in part to number 82, medication shortages.

a. Citizens of the USA demand better quality, fewer side effects, and quicker results. All of these, however, come at a cost. We live in a world where everyone expects prioritization over others. These expectations, then, require more and more studies with more and more potential molecules getting shut down before they get to market. Having more and more potential drugs shut down means the drug development companies need to recoup those losses in the drugs that do end up making it to market. There are dozens of examples of drugs developed decades ago that if introduced now, would never be approved. The side effects and tolerability profiles are such that patients would never allow them.

b. Insurance companies struggle to balance medication affordability for patients with good business acumen. The business of keeping people healthy is a difficult one to balance. A lot of insurance companies are for-profit, so the cost can be a bigger player than patients realize.

c. Independent pharmacies are unable to contract suppliers for the same prices. When there is a large chain or healthcare system, they can create large contracts with the suppliers for lower prices. Small, independent pharmacies can't commit to the same contracts. These added costs, then, are passed to patients. With the overall increase in medication costs already, it can be financially difficult to support local pharmacies.

Tip 84 – Current pharmacy job market is tough

1. Current job market. At the time of this authoring, the field of pharmacy is experiencing a difficult time. Experienced pharmacists are getting laid off to make way for younger, cheaper hires, forcing down salaries. Technicians are hard to find and retain. Pharmacy is not an easy way to make fistfuls of cash the way it used to be. There may be fistfuls of cash, but I assure you, the path is not easy. We're at a pinnacle of increased supply and decreased demand.

a. According to AACP's (American Association of Colleges of Pharmacy[22]) statistics, there were over 62,000 students entering pharmacy school in the fall of 2018. There are 143 colleges of pharmacy. That is a lot of folks entering any field.

Get Involved

Groups

Tip 85 – Join groups

1. Join one group. More than one is great but get in at least one. There are many national, state, and local organizations depending on your area of pharmacy.

    a. APHA/statePhA

        i. APHA = American Pharmacists Association

        ii. This organization works to progress the legislation associated with pharmacy. They work to improve working conditions and scopes of care for pharmacists. They advocated that we can administer immunizations. They have helped the Board of Pharmacy regulating safe working conditions in terms of numbers of pharmacists and technicians working together. They have been advocating for years to get pharmacists the same privileges as nurses, doctors, dentists, and physician's assistants (and others), as legally designated practitioners.

b. ASHP/stateSHP

   i. American Society of Hospital Pharmacists

   ii. This group supports hospital pharmacists by advancing clinical services, providing updates on standards of therapy of commonly hospitalized diseases and illnesses.

   iii. ASHP is the primary organization that provides education for BPS applicants. They have several books and programs available for review.

c. ACCP

   i. American College of Clinical Pharmacists

   ii. As you may guess from the name, this is a group that seeks to advance education and support for developing clinical pharmacists, educators, and students.

d. NCPA

   i. National Community Pharmacists Association

   ii. This organization serves as a voice for independent pharmacy owners and pharmacists.

<u>*Students*</u>

Tip 86 – Work with students and residents

1. Take the time to work with students coming through your workplace. They are the future of the field, and it behooves everyone to ensure they have a great experience and develop strong thought processes.

    a. They are a captive audience that will be looking for jobs soon. You can do your part by showing them the honesty in what your job is. It's also an opportunity to recruit them.

    b. The reason they are there is for us to help sculpt them as practitioners.

    c. Now that you're on the other side of graduation, pass your knowledge to those coming after you. They will be the future once you're gone. If you had a mentor before your journey began, reflect on how valuable it was to have someone you could question and model yourself after.

    d. One example I like to share here involves an experienced pharmacist of about 15 years and a resident on one of his first staffing weekends. It was the three of us. They were working in the main pharmacy, verifying orders, answering phones, and working on new consults. I was in the IV pharmacy overseeing sterile compounding technicians. Both the experienced pharmacist and the new resident came to me frustrated with the other during our shifts. The pharmacist first, frustrated that the resident wasn't prioritizing his work the way she would have liked. Later the resident came to me that the pharmacist was snapping orders at him. I quick wrote a list of roughly what our priorities are, in order, on the weekends, and gave it to him. He immediately adjusted his course of action. When I had a moment, I went back to the pharmacist and explained how I corrected his actions. I reiterated with her that THAT IS WHY RESIDENTS ARE HERE. That's why he is doing a residency, and that is exactly the type of thing he's here to learn. There is a steep learning curve adjusting from being a technician, to being an intern, to a pharmacist. Remember how it felt each time you moved up and help others do the same.

Live Your Life

Tip 87 – Take care of your body

1. This one relates to experience in a broad sense. Regardless of the type of practice you're going into, take care of your body. It is OK to sit down. The number of pharmacists with knee, back, carpal tunnel, and hip problems is mind-blowing. Also, drink water, go to the bathroom, and eat. Take care of your only body.

Tip 88 -Diversify your skills

1. Diversify your skills. If you're interested in computers, there is a huge niche for informatics pharmacists. There are veterinary pharmacists with a passion for animals. There are career coaches that are pharmacists. You can combine almost anything with pharmacy and find a niche for it. Except underwater basket weaving. Maybe that, too. I don't know.

Tip 89 – Balancing life

1. There is no such thing as work/life balance. Balance is static. Balance implies nothing is moving or changing. But that isn't how life works. It is better to seek work/life fulfillment. There will be times in life when it is better to invest your time in work, and times when it is necessary to invest your time at home. Don't sacrifice who you are.

    a. Don't be afraid to take what you perceive to be a lesser role for the sake of your family. If you do, shine in it. You may go far, even if it's not what you wanted. It may not be what you want, but it may be what you need.

    b. One of my pharmacy folks provided the following scenario:

        i. "What is the appropriate time to stay over if your queues are out of control? I know I need to learn to just walk away but when there are over 100 scripts to check, count, or type, I just feel guilty leaving my partner like that. Our pharmacy closes at 9pm and I'm often here until 10pm or later catching up. I have a son who won't truly fall asleep until he knows I'm home safe. I don't want to leave a mess for my partner in the morning. I feel it is not fair to leave a huge mess and start the next day already behind and the cycle starts all over again.

ii. I do have two great partners that stay over for me, too, so it isn't a one-sided situation. I have stayed upwards of 80 hours (honestly stopped counting after that) this year alone. I'm salaried and do not get overtime or even paid for the extra hours I work. We are supposed to cut time that we work over, but that's just a joke and never happens. Our tech hours have been cut like all retail settings and it's flu season. I just can't keep going at this pace (especially without getting paid for it). I work at a very difficult store and the patient population is unforgiving. I get cursed at multiple times a day (and that is not an exaggeration).

iii. I love my job but it's literally killing me and making me question why I even became a pharmacist in the first place. Looking for advice; please be kind."

iv. When I mentioned above that retail metrics are difficult to meet, this is the sort of thing I mean. Alluded to in the Finance Lesson, this is a liability to yourself. Making an error off the clock may not be covered by your employer's malpractice insurance. I reached out to this person repeatedly but didn't hear back. Please don't let this be you. There is an adage that when you die, your job will get posted before your obituary. Make your life mean what you need it to mean.

Lesson 6: Finances

Full disclosure: I am not a financial advisor. But all doctoral (and college in general) programs require acknowledgment of the financial burden undertaken. Twenty years ago, the anticipated forecast of pharmacy careers twenty years out is not what exists today. Twenty years ago, the primary focus was on envisioning what would happen when the Baby Boomer generation began retiring and shifting into nursing homes. They indeed have begun retiring and shifting into nursing homes, but dispensing and pharmaceutical care markets have changed in that time.

Before Pharmacy School

Tip 90 – Look at all costs

1. Look long and hard at those tuition numbers. Awareness is the first step towards making an informed decision. Like undergraduate coursework, masters' and doctoral programs do have in-state and out-of-state tuition differences, but the overall number is higher than undergraduate coursework. Every program has different costs embedded. Don't overlook relocation and the cost of living figures if you'll be moving.

   a. Account for application fees. This amount will vary depending on how many applications you send.

b. Most colleges, once you're accepted, will require a deposit. Some are refundable, and some are not. Most are $500 to $1000.

c. Before classes even start, make sure you've got some cash socked away for your books and supplies. Those are expensive; don't let that surprise you. For some references (books), it may be cheaper to purchase electronic versions than physical versions. As the electronic world continues to expand, expect this to become truer.

d. You may be able to get away without some books. Before you plan on this, try to envision your future practice and what you may want to have physical references for in the future. As discussed at length in numbers 17-18, the areas pharmacists shine in are kinetics and medication delivery. These are unique to pharmacists compared to other healthcare practitioners and may be useful references to keep.

e. Be prepared to dress professionally. Most pharmacy schools will require you to dress professionally for the lab, to most closely mimic the real-world experience. Traditional pharmacy attire is business casual (with exceptions based on site of practice, of course). Make sure you have a few options for meeting with mentors, members of the community, presentations days, lab dress days, etc.

i. Business casual, to be clear, means polo or button-down shirts, long or short sleeve shirts with no words, dress slacks, or skirts. Include white coats here.

ii. Business casual means no to tennis shoes, scrubs, t-shirts, shorts, sweats, or jeans.

During Pharmacy School

Tip 91 – Cost of NAPLEX and MPJE

1. During my second year, one of the upperclassmen mentioned that the NAPLEX and the law exam after graduation, together with the cost of the actual license (note: three separate expenses), all totaled about $1000. As of spring 2019, that number was around $1300 in Minnesota. Research that number in your state. Be mentally, emotionally, and financially prepared for it after graduation.

   a. Be aware you will need to pay annually to keep all licenses updated. The more states you have, the more payments and deadlines you'll have to track.

   b. If you fail these exams, you will need to pay for them again. There's a mandated amount of days before you are eligible for a retake. Currently, it is thirty days for MPJE and forty-five days for NAPLEX.

During Rotations

Tip 92 – Don't forget cost of lunches and parking

1. Some sites may require you to pay for parking while on site. Be prepared for this; ask questions. Other possible costs you may encounter on rotations include lunches. Like the first day of a new job, it's hard to know if it will be easier for you to bring your lunch or plan to eat at work. There is a risk there's no storage for you vs. planning to purchase lunch and realizing they don't have an on-site cafeteria.

Tip 93 – Pay for board exam study aids

1. Do spend money on a high-quality study resource for the NAPLEX. Lots of practice questions.

    a. ASHP publishes a study guide called RxPrep. They are large and in charge and cover practically everything. They aren't as comprehensively as the previous years of school you've just taken, but they are exceptionally thorough. They also have practice questions with answers and explanations.

During Residency or Fellowship

Moonlighting

Tip 94 – Some will allow moonlighting

1. According to ASHP (the accreditation company for residencies), each facility is required to make its own rule about 'moonlighting' (working at a different pharmacy in the evenings or weekends). Residents and even some pharmacists moonlight to bring in extra money. After all, residents ARE licensed pharmacists at this point.

    a. The idea of allowing or disallowing is to prevent burn out and lack of sleep. When this happens, it's more difficult to retain information, which may jeopardize performance and patient care. Disallowing moonlighting also prevents burnout. Burnout is an area getting a lot of attention in healthcare recently.

After Graduation

Tip 95 – Pay student loans ASAP

1. Start repaying your student loans as soon as possible. Don't make the mistake I made. I waited for them to send me a bill or statement that never came. I then defaulted on 21 separate loans. That hurt my credit at a critical time and took a long time to bring it back up. Once you graduate, the

financial institution will give you a six-month grace period before you are required to start paying back your student loans. If you do a residency, this can be income-based (since residents make less than pharmacists), or you can get an extension on your grace period.

a. A lot of new graduates want to pay the minimum and enjoy their newfound financial freedom. Spending this newfound income is understandable, after an extended period of scrimping to get by as a student. Keep in mind that your financial life will only get more complicated. Graduation is typically around the time people start getting married, having kids, and buying a home. You will (normally) be undertaking more and more financial burdens. The earlier you can rid yourself of student loans, the easier.

Tip 96 – Contribute to retirement

1. Contribute to your company's 401k at least the minimum that they match. Contributions are such a small amount, and you won't even notice its absence from your paycheck. It safeguards your retirement.

a. Also recommended: open a Roth IRA.

b. As previously discussed, pharmacy is a volatile profession presently. Having safeguards in place can only help you.

Tip 97 – Pay for malpractice insurance

1. Carry malpractice insurance. It isn't expensive. You are covered at work by your employer to an extent. But anything off protocol (which does happen), any advice you give friends or family, off the clock, and volunteer work will not be covered. Your company's legal team will be more invested in the company's interest over yours. If you are personally sued, your company will not be cover you. HPSO[23], Healthcare Providers Service Organization, is one company that offers malpractice insurance for healthcare providers (not just pharmacists but doctors, nurses, and others as well). Dispensing pharmacists (retail) may have a higher cost than non-dispensing pharmacists.

Lesson 7: Stuck? Additional Reading

StrengthFinder 2.0 by Tom Rath

Tip 98 – Read *StrengthFinder 2.0*

1. I'm going to take a minute and climb up onto my high horse. I adore this research area. The philosophy behind StrengthFinder[24] is not a personality framework but as a peek into how your brain naturally processes the world. Your natural inclinations on how to work through things. My strengths mainly fall into the relationship-building category, which would be of no surprise to anyone who knows me. These may shift somewhat over time (example: a lot of my cohorts had Futuristic as a student, but this fell off after graduation and job acceptance), but for the most part, they stay stable.

    a. Gallup is the research company behind the Strengths. Donald Clifton began the revolution. In this framework, thirty-four different strengths fall into four domains. They were trying to assess what's right with the world, instead of always focusing on negative. They also sought to classify talents. They believe that people naturally possess (or don't possess) a particular talent, but when you add skills, knowledge, and practice, that's how to develop successful people. You can go online to their website and take the quiz. There are two options: your top five strengths only or the entire roster in order. If you get the book, it gives you a code for the quiz (top five only) but then discusses all thirty-four talents and lays out ten actionable items for each, including suggestions for those who have each talent and for working with others who may have that talent. Personally, as a check list-oriented person, I love the action items.

i. Definition of talent: a natural way of thinking, feeling, or behaving.

ii. Definition of strength: the ability to consistently provide near-perfect performance.

iii. "Gallup surveyed more than 10 million people worldwide on the topic of employee engagement (or how positive and productive people are at work), and only one-third "strongly agree" with the statement: "At work, I have the opportunity to do what I do best every day."[24] They have studies to show that people who get to use their top talents at work regularly are more engaged in their work and, therefore, more likely to love their job and less likely to leave.

    1. Engagement is a phenomenal sub-topic, as well!

iv. The first book was Now, Discover Your Strengths, but it was geared primarily towards managers. When Gallup researchers realized how universal the message was, they shifted gears and created this book to fill in the gaps for all.

b. I appreciate this because I feel I'm meant to contribute meaningfully in some way to my field. How can I use what I'm good at to do that? I'm a Developer; it's a natural intuition for me to care for those coming behind me. Once you know your strengths, find ways to use them at work. Use them to discuss your reviews with your manager and develop action plans for moving forward. Using these five strengths will give you purpose and help you feel fulfilled.

    i. Managers may find this information useful when creating teams for new projects. Will the department be initiating a new clinical role? If you speak with someone strong in Strategic or Context, you may be able to anticipate problems on the horizon and avoid them early. Will other departments be wary of this new role or hesitant to accept it? Work with someone strong in Relator or Harmony as a bridge to reach out early and understand the other perspective.

c. There are several podcasts on the topic. One of them, Lead Through Strengths, is hosted by Lisa Cummings. As a Gallup certified Strengths coach, she created a series of thirty-four episodes and highlighted all thirty-four strengths. She discusses ways to highlight your strengths in your CV and opportunities you can look for at work to excel naturally.

d. A person should not focus solely on their strengths. As discussed in number 72, acknowledging weaknesses is important. Like all things in life, the two should be in balance. They even acknowledge this concept in StrengthsFinder 2.0. Knowing your weaknesses, simply the awareness can help one avoid major roadblocks in their life and career. Being able to outsource those necessary details or having a tool (or partner with high strength in areas different from yours) to rely on can be helpful. Awareness is the best place to start.

Tip 99 – If you've already read StrengthFinder 2.0, try...

1. Already read it? Up next...

    a. *First, Break All the Rules*[25]. If you are a manager, (or hope to be one someday), this book is a great follow-up for you. As with our discussion on successful pharmacists, there is no one way for managers to be successful. Because there are as many ways to be a manager as there are managers in the world, Gallup interviewed some of the most successful and well-known managers to study their commonalities.

    b. *Strengths-Based Leadership*[26].

        i. Apparently, you can only be interested in your strengths and seek self-improvement in general if you're seeking management-type positions. The two seem to be perpetually linked. I am here to say it is OK to try and grow personally without seeking management positions.

ii. Managers are people themselves, with their own set of strengths. How they utilize their strengths and draw strengths from the teams they lead can greatly impact their success and the team's success. This book provides tips for optimizing a team as well as continuing the development of your strengths in managerial positions.

c. Emotional Intelligence 2.0[27](EQ). As described by the authors, "the communication between your emotional and rational "brains" is the physical source of emotional intelligence." The idea is to use the rational part of your brain and work WITH the emotional part of your brain; it promotes emotional understanding and awareness. Some people despise the discussion of feelings, but emotions WILL happen to your body, no matter what you do. EQ is a tool to harness that emotion and control your thoughts and body's response, to prevent emotional highjackings.

Indispensable: The Prescription for a Fulfilling Pharmacy Career[28] by Alex Barker, PharmD

Tip 100 – Read *Indispensable*

1. This book is great for preventing professional constipation. This book is also a great "professional enema," as it were. Alex connects to real experience and examples because he IS a real pharmacist. Due to a combination of factors, Alex realized traditional pharmacy was not for him. Thoughts of his own business inspired him. This inspiration pushed him to create his blog, TheHappyPharmD.com[29]. What he finds fulfilling is helping other pharmacists find their path.

   a. His online course, Career Jumpstart is loaded with tools to help with clarity to see your path, resume reviews, salary negotiations, and more.

   b. Alex provides access to real coaching. Alex and his coaches ask the real questions to help you determine what truly is and is not working for you.

   c. This path, in and of itself, is a non-traditional pharmacy option. Alex's business has expanded, and he hires pharmacists as coaches. Connecting back to the StrengthFinder program, people who lead with Developer, Relator, or Individualization may do well in a career path like this.

Atul Gawande

Tip 101 – Read all of Atul Gawande's books

1. All his books are amazing and inspirational. He has a phenomenal way of making his point without shoving it in your face. It's like he's a tour guide carefully guiding you up the Grand Canyon. He's cautious so you won't go too fast and get hurt and at the same time, allows you to see the beauty throughout the climb. After a long, arduous hike, you come to the pinnacle and graciously, miraculously look over everything. And behold the majesty. He doesn't push you into the canyon but holds your hand as its magic meets your eyes. He allows you to understand the magic through your own filter and draw your own conclusions. Atul is a surgeon by trade who also writes books and articles for *The New Yorker*. His several books[30,31][*2] and many articles discuss ways in which we can do better for and by our patients. He discusses fallibility, uncertainty in medicine, and how to make patients feel seen and heard when we don't know what is wrong. He discusses ways we have improved healthcare and how we still have so far to go with widely varied examples like pain, childbirth, and vaccination rates. He was one of the first physicians to acknowledge that end-of-life care and goals are different than during life goals. And that it is OK to talk about these goals with patients and their families.

    a. There's been a lot of research on how best to care for patients when we, as healthcare providers, are mere people. There is still not enough. But Atul has opened the conversation yet again. I am personally grateful for this

---

[*2] Not all inclusive of his work.

conversation. With his array of writings, there are many fantastic quotes to choose from on closing but here is one of my favorites and an area that needs more discussion in pharmacy and healthcare;

i. **"No matter what measures are taken, doctors will sometimes falter, and it isn't reasonable to ask that we achieve perfection. What is reasonable is to ask that we never cease to aim for it."**

Special thanks to...

I cannot thank you properly for all your feedback, inspiration, and support.

Abby Von Ruden, PharmD, BCPS

Blake Tranby-Laudahl, PharmD

Jennifer Coolong, PharmD, BCPS

Million Woldemariam, PharmD

Kristin Kading, PharmD

Klara Janis, PharmD

Kyle Kuczmanski, PharmD

Everyone I work with for tolerating my musings for quite some time.

Every pharmacist, healthcare professional, and person everywhere who inspires me to be better.

References

Lesson one

1. www.usnews.com/education/best-graduate-schools/articles/health-schools-methodology
2. www.pharmacytechnicianguide.com/Best-Pharmacy-Schools.html
3. www.collegeaffordabilityguide.org/subjects/pharmacy/
4. www.collegeaffordabilityguide.org/methodology/
5. www.topuniversities.com/university-rankings/university-subject-rankings/2019/pharmacy-pharmacology
6. www.topuniversities.com/subject-rankings/methodology
7. www.Pharmcas.org
8. http://pcatweb.info/Resources.php
9. www.kaptest.com/pcat/what-is-the-pcat

Lesson four

10. Gilbert, Elizabeth. *Big Magic* (New York, NY: Riverhead Books, 2015).
11. pmp.pharmacy.state.mn.us/
12. www.ashp.org/About-ASHP/Awards/Board-of-Directors-Awards/ASHP-Fellows/FASHP-Guidelines

Lesson five

13. https://nabp.pharmacy/programs/licensure-transfer/
14. Seabright, Mel, PharmD, MBA, "Advice for recent pharmacy school graduates," Pharmacy Times (2015).
    a. www.pharmacytimes.com/contributor/mel-seabright-pharmd-mba/2015/07/advice-for-recent-pharmacy-school-graduates
15. Reiss, Barry, and Gary Hall. *Guide to Federal Pharmacy Law 9th Edition* (Boyton Beach, FL: Apothecary Press, 2016).
16. www.deadiversion.usdoj.gov/pubs/manuals/pharm2/pharm_manual.pdf
17. www.deadiversion.usdoj.gov/schedules/index.html
18. https://nabp.pharmacy/programs/naplex/
19. https://nabp.pharmacy/programs/mpje/
20. www.hhs.gov/hipaa/index.html
21. Fields, Jonathan. Uncertainty: Turning Fear and Doubt into Fuel for Brilliance (Portfolio, 2012)
22. www.aacp.org/article/academic-pharmacys-vital-statistics

Lesson six

23. www.HPSO.com

Lesson seven

24. Rath, Tom. *Strengths Finder 2.0* (New York, NY: Gallup Press, 2007).
25. Buckingham, Marcus. *First, Break All the Rules: What the World's Greatest Managers Do Differently* (New York, NY: Simon & Schuster, 1999).
26. Rath, Tom, and Conchie, Barry. *Strengths Based Leadership* (New York, NY: Gallup Press, 2008).
27. Bradberry, Travis, and Greaves, Jean. *Emotional Intelligence 2.0* (San Deigo, CA: TalentSmart, 2009).
28. Barker, Alex. Indispensable (Mandala Tree Publishing, 2019).
29. www.TheHappyPharmD.com
30. Gawande, Atul. *Complications: A Surgeon's Notes on an Imperfect Science* (New York, NY: Picador, 2002).
31. Gawande, Atul. *Better: A Surgeon's Notes on Performance* (New York, NY: Picador 2007).

About the Expert

Ann Klemz, PharmD, is a hospital pharmacist from Minnesota. She graduated from the University of Minnesota, Duluth campus in 2012.

She has worked in the field of pharmacy as a technician, intern, and pharmacist for over twenty years. She's worked in retail, hospital, minor clinical roles, home infusion, and hospice. Her perspective is inclusive and unique.

Her strengths include Harmony, Adaptability, Developer, Empathy, and Positivity, with a punch of Activator and Intellection for good measure.

When she's not at work, she can be found drinking coffee, cross-stitching, and mitigating the craziness of her three-child household with her loving partner, Tim.

HowExpert publishes quick 'how to' guides on all topics from A to Z by everyday experts. Visit HowExpert.com to learn more.

Recommended Resources

- HowExpert.com – Quick 'How To' Guides on All Topics by Everyday Experts.
- HowExpert.com/books – HowExpert Books
- HowExpert.com/products – HowExpert Products
- HowExpert.com/courses – HowExpert Courses
- HowExpert.com/clothing – HowExpert Clothing
- HowExpert.com/membership – Learn All Topics from A to Z by Real Experts.
- HowExpert.com/affiliates – HowExpert Affiliate Program
- HowExpert.com/jobs – HowExpert Jobs
- HowExpert.com/writers – Write About Your #1 Passion/Knowledge/Expertise.
- YouTube.com/HowExpert – Subscribe to HowExpert YouTube.
- Instagram.com/HowExpert – Follow HowExpert on Instagram.
- Facebook.com/HowExpert – Follow HowExpert on Facebook.

Printed in Great Britain
by Amazon